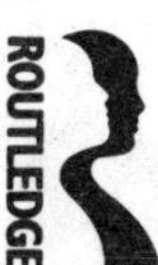

London and New York

First published 1975 by Unwin Hyman Ltd
Second edition 1980
Third edition 1986
Second impression 1990

Reprinted 1992 and 1993
by Routledge
11 New Fetter Lane, London EC4P 4EE

Simultaneously published in the USA and Canada
by Routledge
29 West 35th Street, New York, NY 10001

Printed and bound in Great Britain by
Biddles Ltd, Guildford and King's Lynn

British Library Cataloguing in Publication Data
Pringle, Mia Kellmer
The needs of children. – 3rd ed.
1. Child psychology
I. Title
155.4 BF721

Library of Congress Cataloging in Publication Data available

ISBN 0–415–08392–3

Contents

Introduction to the Third Edition

Mia Kellmer Pringle died in 1983; but this, one of the most popular of her books, is as relevant today as it was when she wrote it in 1975. For the second edition in 1980, research findings were updated and new items added to the bibliography, and the same procedure has been followed for this edition. Over forty new references have been added; a few passages have been revised to reflect current thinking or take account of new research. Otherwise the message of the book remains unchanged.

Mia Pringle used the pronoun 'he' to refer to the child throughout. We have become more sensitive to this usage, but to avoid clumsiness it has been retained.

Thanks are due to Ken Fogelman, Jean Seglow and Doria Pilling for their help with this revision. Ronald Davie, who was the editor for the original book, was able to act in a similar capacity for this revision, thus ensuring continuity.

ROSEMARY DINNAGE

Introduction to the Second Edition

During the past forty years there has been a virtual revolution in children's physical development: they are taller, they mature earlier, certain diseases have been almost eliminated, and obesity is a more serious problem than malnutrition. It had been hoped that rising standards of physical health and material prosperity would reduce the incidence of educational backwardness, maladjustment and delinquency. However, it has become increasingly evident that problems of emotional, social and educational malfunctioning will not be solved by improvements in standards of living alone; these make satisfactory family and community life more likely but do not ensure it. Yet few would deny that there is much room for improvement at a time when vandalism, violence, drug addiction and crime are causing widespread concern.

So far, little systematic attempt has been made to raise the general level of emotional and social resilience. A first step in this direction would be to bring together available insights from the many relevant fields to present a coherent picture of the present state of knowledge about children's needs. The purpose of this book is an attempt to do so. Though based on research findings, it has been written in as jargon-free and non-technical a style as possible. It aims to be a source document for those who wish to inform themselves about what is known regarding child development and parenthood as well as those who will be concerned with disseminating such knowledge. Thus, it should interest students of education, social work and medicine, as well as policy-makers and intelligent laymen, especially parents.

HOW THE BOOK CAME TO BE WRITTEN

It was commissioned by the British Government's Department of Health and Social Security. The terms of reference were as follows:

> To prepare a comprehensive document about the developmental needs of all children, about the ways in which these needs are normally met, and about the consequences for the emotional, intellectual, social and physical growth and development of children when, for one reason or another, these needs are not adequately met.

The book is based on my own experience and knowledge of working with children and their families, as well as my personal research work; I have also drawn extensively on the results of the Bureau's studies, undertaken under my direction. To make the task of writing it somewhat more manageable in the six months stipulated by the Department, I decided to confine myself to conditions in developed Western societies; to place the main emphasis on children's psycho-social needs; and to devote relatively greater attention to the development and needs of the younger age groups. Throughout, the convention of using 'he' to include 'she' has been followed to avoid the rather clumsy 's/he' or the constant repetition of 'he or she'.

At the same time as commissioning the writing of this book, the Department also asked the Bureau to undertake a complementary literature review. This was published in 1978 entitled *Controversial Issues in Child Development* (Elek Books).

In the second edition of *The Needs of Children* I have not only taken into account the findings reported in the above literature review but I have also incorporated new results from, and given new references to, research reported between 1976 and 1979. In addition, certain sections have been expanded.

THE NATIONAL CHILD DEVELOPMENT STUDY (1958 COHORT)

Since I draw to quite a large extent on the findings from the Bureau's largest project, the National Child Development Study, a description of its overall design and aims might be of help.

In 1958, for the purpose of a Perinatal Mortality Survey, information was gathered on virtually every baby born in England, Scotland and Wales during the week 3–9 March. This group of children – numbering some 17,000 births in all – is therefore a completely representative cross section; the term 'cohort' has been coined for such groups.

An unparalleled amount of sociological, obstetric and medical information was collected concerning the mother, the course of pregnancy and labour. In addition, a great deal of detailed information was amassed on her baby at the time of birth and within the first few weeks of life.

Subsequently, the National Children's Bureau embarked on a long-term, multi-disciplinary follow-up investigation of all the children in this birth week. This project is called the National Child Development Study (1958 cohort). So far, follow-ups have been undertaken when the subjects were seven, eleven, sixteen and twenty-three years old. On each occasion, very extensive information is gathered from four main sources: schools provide a comprehensive picture of each pupil's attainment, behaviour and adjustment as well as information about the school itself; secondly, each mother, and sometimes the father too, is interviewed to obtain details about the home environment as well as about the child's development and behaviour; thirdly, data are gathered on each child's height, weight, speech, hearing, vision and motor co-ordination, all obtained in a special medical examination; fourthly, a number of attainment tests and other assessments are completed by each child.

It is planned to continue studying the growth and development of the children at least until they have reached adulthood and have themselves become parents, because the project provides an unrivalled opportunity to find answers to many important questions which are neither known nor easy to discover by other means. Three of these deserve to be singled out. First, by looking at a large representative group at various ages, it becomes possible to describe and make generalisations about their health, physical development and home environment, as well as about their behaviour and educational attainments. This provides a base line against which the parent, teacher, doctor or psychologist can judge the development and needs of a particular child; while the policy-maker and administrator can judge the effectiveness and adequacy of existing services in the light of the conditions which are revealed.

Second, the development of special groups of children, such as the handicapped, the exceptionally gifted or those born illegitimate, can be compared with that of the whole cohort, and factors affecting their needs and performance, both adverse and beneficial, can be identified. Third, the development of all the children can be examined longitudinally. This makes it possible to unravel the interrelationship between social, medical and obstetric factors in the mother, the baby's birth history and ante-natal development on the one hand, and the child's subsequent all-round growth and adjustment, on the other. For example, a picture can be built up of the long-term relationships between parental social background, low birth weight and the child's level of educational achievements. Or the growing child's family and social background can be assessed and it can be established how many children who showed behaviour difficulties at the age of seven years, still do so at eleven and sixteen years; and in what ways they and their environments differ from those of children who have 'outgrown' them in the intervening years; as well as from those who developed behaviour difficulties only at the age of eleven or sixteen years.

Thus each successive follow-up provides valuable, descriptive and normative material about a representative group of British children at a particular age, showing not only their level of development but also the relationship between various stages of and factors affecting growth. In addition, and possibly even more valuable, the longitudinal nature of the whole project makes it possible to study changes in development of the same children over a period of time.

THE BRITISH EDUCATIONAL SCENE

A word of explanation may be helpful to explain allusions in the text. Education in Britain is compulsory for all children from five to sixteen years of age. It is provided free of charge in 'maintained' schools for which local education authorities, and ultimately the Department of Education and Science, are responsible. In fact, about 20 per cent of children start school before their fifth birthday although some may do so only on a part-time basis; and about 25 per cent stay on voluntarily after the age of sixteen years. From five years onwards, they have to attend five days a week for about seven hours (9.00 A.M. to 4.00 P.M.). During the lunchtime break, a cooked meal is available for those whose parents wish them to have it; for children of poor families, this is provided free of charge.

Primary school education covers the age from five to eleven years followed by secondary schooling from eleven to sixteen and beyond. In some areas, a new division has developed, namely first schools from five to nine years; middle schools from nine to twelve or thirteen years; and secondary education from then on. The more prevalent primary school pattern consists of two parts: infant schools which children attend for two or three years, according to when their birthday falls, and junior schools from seven to eleven. The number of children in a class has been slowly but steadily falling over the past fifty years. It is considered by teachers that in the primary schools, thirty children should be regarded as a reasonable maximum, but at present about 10 per cent of children are still in classes of more than forty pupils.

Infant schools have more in common with the aims and organisation of nursery schools than with later stages of schooling. Progressive methods whereby children learn by discovery, by active participation, and at a rate appropriate to their age and stage of development, are the rule in the majority of such schools. Quite a few junior schools continue this method of teaching. However, many more prefer the older, traditional, more formal methods of instruction because most head teachers are not convinced that children learn effectively by these newer, child-centred ways.

Secondary schools have also been changing their organisation and curriculum, although these changes have been slower and less widespread. At the same time, selection at the age of eleven years to 'cream-off' the most able 20 per cent of children to go to grammar schools, is being replaced by the introduction of a system of comprehensive schools. In England about 80 per cent and in Scotland and Wales over 90 per cent of all eleven-year-olds were receiving their secondary education in such schools in 1978.

For the under-fives, education may be provided in nursery schools devoted entirely to children from two to five years, and in nursery classes which are attached to primary schools. In addition, local education authorities are obliged to carry out examinations and to provide special educational treatment for children from the age of two years where the presence of a handicap is known or suspected. Some handicapped children, such as the blind or deaf, may be admitted to special schools from the age of two years.

At present, nursery school education is available only to a minority of under-fives, some 10 per cent overall. This proportion varies from one part of the country to another and also between social groups – for example, only 2.5 per cent of the children of unskilled manual workers attend nursery schools, compared with 22.5 per cent of those whose fathers are managers.

Widespread dissatisfaction over the shortage of places in nursery schools and classes led to one of the most successful self-help organisations set up by parents during the past twenty years. This is the Pre-School Playgroups Association. Established almost single-handed in 1962, by a mother of young children, it had ten years later produced over 7,000 local groups catering for more than 200,000 children between the ages of two and five years. By 1982, there were over 12,000 local groups catering for over 400,000 pre-school children, including toddlers, and this despite a falling birth-rate. These playgroups are run largely by mothers themselves on a rota basis, a small fee being charged for each child to cover the cost of equipment and overhead expenses. By now, over half of the groups have a qualified supervisor. Inevitably, children from middle-class homes make greater use of this facility, not least because the concept of active maternal involvement has continued to be the major principle – a principle less readily translated into practice in working-class areas.

The Association's rapid growth clearly demonstrates that it is meeting a real need. Indeed, twice as many children now attend playgroups as are in nursery schools and classes. While increasing financial support is being given to them both by central and local government, the nursery school world has adopted a somewhat suspicious, if not hostile, attitude. This voluntary self-help movement is seen as a threat to the professionally trained nursery school teacher. Added to the fear of 'dilution of labour' by amateurs is the concern lest playgroups weaken the case for more nursery school provision.

MIA KELLMER PRINGLE

Acknowledgments

While many people gave generous help, any omissions, weaknesses or inconsistencies which remain are mine alone.

First, I must thank the Department of Health and Social Security who sponsored the writing of this book. Next, four 'official readers' were invited jointly by the Department and myself to comment on the text. They were Professors David Donnison, Michael Rutter, Gordon Trasler and Bill Wall. I am deeply grateful for their constructive criticisms which led to many improvements.

A number of friends and colleagues also offered to read the manuscript. In particular, I am grateful to Mrs L. A. Hersov, Mr A. Jacka, Mrs S. Kitzinger, Mr and Mrs A. Rampton, Miss J. Rowe, Baroness Serota and Dame Eileen Younghusband for their helpful suggestions.

All my colleagues at the National Children's Bureau were offered the opportunity to comment on the manuscript. Their assistance was much appreciated, particularly that of Miss D. Birchall, Professor R. Davie, and Dr R. Pearson.

Invaluable support and encouragement were given to me by my husband, Len Hooper, throughout the period of writing, re-writing and checking the final proofs. He read and re-read every draft, commenting critically and constructively on matters of both substance and detail. If the book is judged to be intelligible to a lay readership then a great deal of the credit must go to him in helping me to make it so.

MIA KELLMER PRINGLE

September 1979

1. Some Basic Concepts

Children's physical, emotional, social and intellectual needs must all be met if they are to enjoy life, develop their full potential and grow into participating, contributing adults. At present only physical needs are being satisfactorily met, at least to any considerable extent. Hence, the main emphasis in this book will be on psycho-social needs.

Five basic premises underlie the discussion and these are briefly outlined in this section. They are: that the environment is of overriding importance; that it is the early years of life which are particularly vital to later development; that there are marked individual differences in the extent and pace of children's growth; that vast improvements could be brought about in their emotional, social, intellectual and educational achievements; and that the strategy so successfully used in the health field may well be appropriate also to these aspects of development.

THE NATURE-NURTURE ISSUE

The first premise is that, for all practical purposes of social action and policy, the environment is of overriding importance. Human capacity to learn is such that the new-born child can adapt to widely different environments. Since, to begin with, he has a rather limited range of innate behavioural mechanisms, this very limited capacity makes him entirely dependent on his environment: having only the potential for becoming human, he must needs have a human environment to do so.

This is clearly shown by two phenomena; first, by the extremely circumscribed development of children who lack the necessary sense organs to perceive, communicate and interact with their environment, such as the deaf-blind (Helen Keller being the most famous example of success in overcoming these obstacles); secondly, by the fortunately rare cases of children who spent their early years in extreme isolation: by the time they were rescued, aged six years or more, they had acquired few truly 'human' characteristics. The same need for an appropriately nurturing environment is illustrated by the fact that even great gifts, such as the ability to compose music, might not be realised, or even discovered, in a culture without music.

Somewhat less extreme examples of the environment's overriding influence relate to sex-typing – the teaching of the socially expected sex role – which normally begins at birth. One of the first questions asked about a baby is whether it is a boy or a girl and from then onwards parental attitudes and expectations become different according to the answer given: both in major and minor ways, the child will be treated, and expected to behave, differently. Clothes, toys, subtle differences in words, play, hugs, rewards, punishments and parental example, surround the child with a world which clearly distinguishes behaviour expected from boys and girls.

Those psychological characteristics considered appropriate will be developed by about the third year of life; and throughout childhood the 'assigned' sex role will be practised in social relations, in play and in fantasy, and be continually reinforced by the responses and expectations of others. Finally, it will be reinforced at puberty by the various physiological changes.

In the past, the consistency and reliability of the sex role performance had been thought to be due to its innate basis. Now many studies have shown the immense influence of psychological and social factors in determining sexual attitudes and behaviour. Furthermore, studies of children born with the same defect of physical sexual development have illustrated that they can be raised either as boys or as girls. With very few exceptions, they grew up to behave in accordance with the sex role to which they had been – almost arbitrarily – assigned (Hampson and Hampson, 1961; Kagan and Moss, 1962; Money, 1963; Maccoby and Jacklin, 1975).

These findings suggest that children learn to behave in 'masculine' or 'feminine' ways through being treated as such; in other words, the gender role is psychologically determined first by parental and then by wider society's expectations.

This conclusion is in line with other findings relating to educational achievement. These showed the influence of parental attitudes and expectations on scholastic progress (Douglas, 1964 and 1968; Seginer, 1983). Other studies have demonstrated that children 'demoted' to lower streams were soon conforming to the lower standards prevailing in them (Lunn, 1970; Brophy, 1983).

There is another developmental area where this is still a controversial issue, namely the question of the relative contribution made to intellectual development by the genes and the environment respectively. This has been debated, with greater or lesser heat, for many years. Following Jensen's much-quoted article, it is still a topical controversy (Vernon, 1979; Eysenck and Kamin, 1981; Taylor, 1981).

The current debate differs in two ways from that which raged in the 1930s. On the one hand, few would now deny that environment plays a part in shaping a child's intelligence, even if they believe heredity to have a much greater influence; the pure environmentalist has been discredited too. On the other hand, more explicit racial implications have now been added to the previous political overtones. This has increased the bitterness of the argument as well as its implications for current political and educational thinking.

Though a belief in the interaction of heredity and environment is the most generally accepted standpoint, available research findings allow a wide range of possible interpretations. The debate about measuring the relative importance of the two is likely to remain rather sterile, since it is doubtful whether conclusive evidence can ever be provided. This situation is only too familiar to the farmer: to obtain a good crop of wheat, he needs not only good seed but also good soil and appropriate moisture, temperature and fertiliser to nourish its growth. However, all of these can be controlled and varied in a way which would be neither acceptable, nor indeed at present possible, in relation to the genetic and environmental components of human beings.

Yet the mistaken belief about reliable measurement is most clearly shown in relation to the I.Q. The credibility of most educational testing – whether concerned with assessing attainments, aptitudes or intelligence – depends largely on a tautology: the validity of the tests is demonstrated by their ability to predict performance at school; yet such performance amounts to an ability to perform well on tasks similar to those in the tests. This has led to the false impression that doing well in tests necessarily means a greater competence in coping, later on, with life in general. Hence there is a 'grave danger of perpetuating a mythological meritocracy' (McClelland, 1973).

The solution is not – as some would have it – simply to abandon testing; if for no other reason than that subjective judgements are considerably less reliable. Instead, three changes are required: first, the search for innate factors, such as intelligence, should be abandoned to be replaced by measuring instead improvement resulting from new experiences and from deliberate teaching. Secondly, currently used items, consisting of very artificial word and number games should be replaced by issues and problems occurring in everyday social and occupational life. Thirdly, rate of progress over time should become the yardstick for learning potential instead of the static concept of the I.Q.

Genetic-environmental interaction starts in utero and hence 'pure' inborn abilities and characteristics can never be assessed. For example, the development of the nervous system in the foetus and new-born is affected during pregnancy and parturition by adverse conditions, e.g., malnutrition or exposure to certain diseases, heavy manual work, smoking, drug-taking or extreme anxiety. Thus a child may be born with a brain which is incapable of normal development, not because of defective genes but because of pre-natal conditions or birth injury. On the other hand, inborn temperamental differences inevitably affect the environment; for example, a hypersensitive, irritable baby is likely to call out irritability in his mother which in turn only serves to increase his own irritability.

> In growth of all kinds, the interaction of powerful genetic forces and powerful environmental forces is at work cumulatively over long periods of development. In optimum environments, genetic factors will appear predominant and environment will appear less important because its influence is roughly constant. In sub-optimum environments, environmental effects will appear more obvious (Clarke and Clarke, 1972).

The weight or influence exerted solely by the nurturing process could only be determined by a study of identical twins who alone are perfectly matched genetically. However, ethical reasons preclude the deliberate and extreme environmental manipulation which would be needed to make possible a systematic exploration of the effects of very different experiences on subsequent development.

There is one well-documented and detailed study of two pairs of identical twins who were reared apart from early infancy and did not meet again until they were in their late twenties (Hudson, 1970).

The two girls had been adopted into very different homes and hence their upbringing and education had also been markedly different. By the age of thirty-five, there were even marked physical differences: the one who had had the much easier life was, for example, better preserved, apparently physiologically younger and an inch taller; there were also marked differences in ability, attainments, personality and overt behaviour. The two boys, on the other hand, were adopted by families who were of absolutely the same social and economic status and these twins led extremely parallel lives. By adulthood, the similarities between them were quite striking in almost all areas of development and physically they had repeatedly been mistaken for each other by strangers.

No doubt the controversy regarding the relative contribution of heredity and environment (including the intra-uterine) to children's abilities, attainments and adjustment will continue. That genetic and physical factors play some role, if only in setting limits to potential development, is widely accepted. At the same time, all available evidence confirms that, from a practical viewpoint, the most important element in shaping behaviour and development is the environment in general and other people in particular. Hence, from the point of view of action – whether preventive or remedial – this is where intervention should be concentrated.

> Genetics, after all, describes only the raw material on which a particular culture acts. As educational systems evolve, so too do the skills of the individuals within them. Logically, we can set limits to children's capacity to learn only if every permutation of their environment, every method of nurturing and teaching them, has been exhausted. This is a task we have scarcely begun; and which, even in principle, we could never finish (Hudson, 1972).

EARLY EXPERIENCE, DEVELOPMENTAL PACE AND SENSITIVE PERIODS

Longitudinal research is beginning to provide an understanding of the pattern of human growth. Three quite specific features have emerged which have important practical implications for child rearing. First, the development of various basic characteristics does not proceed in equal units per unit of time, i.e., growth does not take place at an even pace.

Secondly, for most aspects, the period of most rapid growth takes place in the early years (i.e., from conception to six years or so) and is then followed by periods of less and less rapid growth with a 'spurt' at puberty; for some characteristics there is as much quantitative growth in a single year of a child's life as there is in eight to ten years at other stages in his development.

Thirdly, available evidence suggests that environmental influences have the greatest effect during the most rapid periods of growth. From this it follows that it is experiences and opportunities during the early years of life which are particularly vital to later development. This is the second basic principle adopted in this document.

A few examples are given as illustrations. These are drawn from the Bureau's National Child Development Study (see NCDS User Support Group, 1985); the Berkeley Growth Study (Bayley, 1964); the longitudinal studies of the Fels Institute (Kagan and Moss, 1962); the writer's own research; and the evidence synthesised by Bloom (1964).

Physical development

Height is the most extreme case of the first generalisation referred to above. During the nine months from conception to birth, growth is of the same absolute magnitude as it is during the nine years from three to twelve; and from conception to the age of about two and a half years, half the full adult stature is attained. The brain's weight doubles during the first year of life while during the next nineteen years increasing by only one and a half times (Brierley, 1976). Hence, one would expect that it is pre-natally and during early infancy that the environment has the greatest effect, for better or worse.

Intellectual development

As much development takes place in the first four years of life as in the following thirteen years. It has been estimated that about 50 per cent of intellectual growth takes place between conception and the fourth year, and about 30 per cent between the ages of four to eight years. Unlike physical development, however, it continues well into adulthood, but the pace becomes very much slower after eighteen years or thereabouts.

With regard to vocabulary, by eight years of age, about 50 per cent of the level attained by eighteen years will have been reached.

So again, early environmental influences have a marked effect on measurable cognitive functioning. Recent studies suggest that social class differences, affecting language development, emerge during the first year of life and become unequivocal by about the age of three (Kagan, 1971).

Emotional and social development

Precise and objective evidence remains very inadequate in this area. Paradoxically, less is known about the development of normal than of deprived, disturbed or delinquent children. Two aspects of personality have, however, received particular attention, partly because of their central significance in personal relations and partly because they are more readily observable than other characteristics. These are aggressiveness and dependence on others for support and direction.

Differences between boys and girls in the development of these aspects can be noted early and the 'sex-appropriate' behaviour becomes well established during the pre-school years. This suggests that for personality development, too, the early years are of great importance.

With regard to behaviour and adjustment, problems are already apparent among children in infant schools, by which age some 14 per cent show considerable difficulties in school (Chazan, Laing and Jackson, 1971; Pringle et al., 1966). The lower the parental occupational status, the lower tends to be the proportion of well-adjusted children (Davie et al., 1972).

Educational development

Available evidence suggests that of a child's general attainment at the age of eighteen, approximately half has been reached when he is about nine years old. However, the capacity to respond to, and benefit from, education inevitably depends on the level of a child's intellectual, language and emotional maturity. Therefore, it is again experience during the pre-school years which has a vital influence on later scholastic progress.

Findings from the National Child Development Study show that even as early as the age of seven years there are marked differences in scholastic attainments between children coming from each of the five occupational groups into which the Census divides the total population; during the following four years, these differences in attainment continue to widen (Fogelman and Goldstein, 1976). With regard to children removed from their families, their educational difficulties were found to be more severe, the earlier the child's first separation from home and the less contact his parents had maintained with him subsequently.

Differential growth, which takes place during early childhood, is presented below in summarised form for the six aspects of development just discussed. It is based on the assumption that growth is more or less complete by the age of eighteen to twenty years. What is shown is the age by which – according to Bloom's synthesis of available knowledge – the half-way stage of development is reached for each aspect.

	Age in years
Height (from conception)	2½
Intelligence	4
Vocabulary	8
Aggressiveness in boys	3
Dependence in girls	4
School attainments	9

'Sensitive' periods

It is evident then that normally more progress, change and development take place during the first few years of life than in any comparable time thereafter. This is true too of the post-natal growth of the brain itself, which is more rapid in the first two years. In the case of young birds and mammals, the existence of 'sensitive' and 'critical' periods over a very wide range of development is incontrovertibly established; during these periods, there is greatly heightened susceptibility to specific experiences, such as stimulation or isolation, which may have a lasting and irreversible effect.

Whether in children's development there are also such 'sensitive' periods during which responsiveness to the environment is maximal – and hence learning optimal – has not been quite so clearly demonstrated. The evidence suggests they do occur but that they are not as 'critical' or fixed as, say, the result of 'imprinting' is in birds. However, there are definite indications that children, too, respond more readily to various environmental opportunities at certain periods: strong emotional relationships, particularly with their mothers, are developed during the first twenty-four months; and skills such as walking and talking are usually acquired at roughly similar ages by most children. Conversely, if a child has not learned to speak at all by the age of five years or to read by the age of ten (despite normal opportunities to do so and in the absence of sensory handicaps), then it is most unlikely that quite normal speech or reading ability will ever be achieved.

At the same time, not only are these sensitive or optimal periods of longer duration among the human young but also later learning can and does take place, although it is slower and more difficult then.

That early childhood experiences have great potency is quite beyond doubt; so is the fact that their consequences are often long-lasting and may be very difficult to alter. Of course, experiences later in a child's life may also have a similarly marked or lasting effect on subsequent development.

Reversibility and recovery

As in most other fields, prevention is undoubtedly better than cure. Hence, the attention and emphasis now being given to the earliest years, indeed months, of life is entirely justified. What is not justified is any pessimism which has followed, either from work on 'sensitive' periods or from recent, only partly successful, attempts to reverse the effects of a deprived early environment.

This pessimism has a three-fold basis: first, the growing evidence that the effects of early disadvantage or deprivation are multiple and cumulative; secondly, that the provision of more educational opportunities during the past twenty-five years has least benefited those most in need of them; and thirdly, the apparently disappointing long-term results produced by pre-school intervention programmes, such as Headstart in the USA.

In fact, the first and second arguments are linked. The belief that formal education could itself bring about the desired changes can now be seen to have been unrealistic in the light of more recent understanding of the nature of emotional, social and intellectual development. With regard to intervention programmes, those devised so far have all been too short-term; they have been further handicapped by too narrow a framework, too late a start, too limited a methodology and insufficient theoretical knowledge about early learning. Also, most of them failed to involve the parents; there is now some evidence that concurrent maternal participation can lead to substantial improvement (Halsey, 1972; Midwinter, 1972). Recent evaluations are in fact more positive.

In fact, there is cause for optimism regarding the possibility of recovery and reversibility of even severe and early deprivation. First, work with mentally subnormal patients over the past fifteen years has shown that some degree of recovery can be achieved even in adulthood (Clarke and Clarke, 1978).

The second source of evidence comes from the study of children who have suffered prolonged and extremely severe social isolation in early life. Unfortunately, in most of these cases, their subsequent history has been inadequately documented. Inevitably, what happened during the period of isolation could only be pieced together retrospectively; also, details of the rehabilitation process itself have been inadequate but for a few exceptions (Mason, 1942; Davis, 1947; Koluchova, 1972). These suggest that considerable improvement, if not complete recovery, is possible, given a carefully devised and prolonged programme of rehabilitation.

When labour was cheap, and fulfilment of potential the prerogative of a minority, waste of human abilities was not seen as a problem. Now this is fortunately no longer so. A beginning has been made with exploring systematically both available and new psychological, educational and social methods for preventing or reducing the loss of human potential; and for undoing and, if possible, reversing the effects of early neglect or damage.

INDIVIDUAL DIFFERENCES

In the physical field, it is readily accepted that large individual differences may exist, even among children in one family. When a healthy, well-nourished child is nevertheless of small stature and rather slight build, this may cause comment, even regret perhaps, but neither concern nor reproach. Although theoretically there is a similar understanding in regard to intellectual, educational, emotional and social development, yet in practice, parents, and to some extent professional workers too, react with less tolerance and understanding.

Slow intellectual and educational progress are readily attributed to 'laziness' with disapproval and punishment being meted out in the hope of bringing about improvement. A similar attitude is taken to emotional and social 'deviation', such as timidity or shyness. This then is the third basic principle: that there are as marked individual differences in the extent and pace of children's intellectual, education, emotional and social development, as there are of physical development.

Recent evidence indicates how very early individual differences in behaviour and 'cognitive style' can be observed. 'New-born infants write their signature with their sucking rhythm, showing a constant individual pattern in the number of sucks and intervals between sucks per minute' (Lipsitt, 1972). Though this is congenitally determined, nevertheless the baby learns very quickly to modify his sucking pattern in response to the way he is fed.

The next example of early individual differences shows the equally early interaction between nature and nurture: 'Stable individual differences were found in motor activity [of new-borns] both in hospital and at home... The mothers of the more active infants were more demonstrative towards their children and appeared to form a stronger and earlier attachment to the baby' (Campbell, 1972). Here is the beginning of an egg-and-chicken question: a more active baby probably calls out stronger maternal feelings and a more 'motherly' mother is likely to encourage the baby to be more active and responsive.

A third example of individual differences relates to the respective development of boys and girls (Seward and Seward, 1981). Considerable evidence shows boys to be much more variable and vulnerable from birth onwards. For example, their morbidity and their accident rate is generally higher; their speech, language development and level of reading attainment are poorer, at least during the first ten years of life; a much higher proportion show emotional and behaviour difficulties, ranging from enuresis and school phobia to delinquency and crime; the majority of drop outs are also male. Girls, on the other hand, 'are born with slightly more mature skeletal and nervous systems and gradually increase their developmental lead (in absolute terms) throughout childhood' (Tanner, 1974).

Various hypotheses have been put forward to account for these sex differences. Most suggest a combination of and interaction between genetic, biological and environmental factors. Some consider that boys' greater deviancy may be a function of a Y chromosome and hence largely genetically determined (Birley, 1973). Cultural, social and family influences are stressed by others and motivational aspects are also thought to play a part; for example, most parents are more ambitious career-wise for boys than girls. On the other hand, fathers cannot so readily serve as models for their sons; not only do most of them spend the major part of the child's waking life away from home, but also they do work which their sons can neither observe nor clearly comprehend. Also, in Western society a boy is expected to be more active, outgoing, aggressive and less home-centred – not only in childhood but in his future work and leisure interests too – than a girl. Peers too exert greater pressures on boys than girls by their competitive self-assertiveness, in particular in relation to games and physical prowess. Additionally, the roles which boys are expected to play are less consistent than those demanded of girls: for example, the greater stress laid on boys' educational progress means that they must be more studious and intellectual which inevitably conflicts with being more active physically and more outgoing; also physical prowess is not necessarily allied to educational abilities. Such conflicting expectations may to some extent at least account for the greater deviancy found among boys. Though all these expectations may now be changing, or at least becoming modified, such change is unlikely to bring rapid results.

It follows that methods of child-rearing must take individual differences more into account than at present. The practical implications would seem to be three-fold. First, only a few directions or antidotes can be of universal application; and it is the quality of understanding – often intuitive, rarely fully explicit – which can best guide parents in applying their knowledge of developmental needs to the upbringing of a particular child. An understanding of his physical and mental equipment at any given stage, and hence his readiness at a given time to respond and to adapt, is the most reliable gauge of whether parental expectations are appropriate. From a general knowledge of the principles of child-rearing parents need to fashion a method 'tailor-made' for each particular child at each particular stage of his development and suited to his particular environment.

The second implication is that it is never possible to treat two children in the same family alike if the aim is to treat each appropriately. Nor is 'the same family' psychologically the same for each child: partly because of the interaction between the parents' personalities and that of the child; partly because the family constellation itself is different in respect of each member of the family – the parents' age and the child's position in the family (first-born, middle one, etc.) are just two examples.

The third implication lies in making allowance for the fact that just as physical endowment ranges from the resilient to the delicate, so children differ genetically in their intellectual and emotional constitution and susceptibility to stress. At the same time, environmental influences come into play at birth and in some respects from conception onwards; and they have potentially a far greater effect than has hitherto been generally realised.

THE POSSIBILITY OF IMPROVEMENT

While no-one would question that it is possible to bring about vast improvements in children's physical health and educational achievements, there is less agreement in relation to intelligence and still outright scepticism about emotional and social aspects. Nor is there agreement about how any such improvement might be brought about. Nevertheless, that the possibility exists in all these areas is the fourth basic assumption made in this book.

One reason for doubt may be that much more is known about deficiencies and failure than about 'optimal' or even normal growth. For example, there have been many studies of delinquent children or poor readers but there is little detailed understanding of how language or reading skills are acquired; or, even more important, what enables a child to develop normally despite an adverse emotional or social environment.

The whole issue is further complicated by the fact that society rarely asks – and certainly has no answer to – the question: into what kind of people do we want today's children to grow? Even to pose the question could give a new slant both to child-rearing methods and to research.

Physical development

The past forty years or so have seen in this country what amounts to a revolution in children's health: they are taller; they mature earlier; and certain diseases have been virtually eliminated (Tanner, 1974).

Even so, there remains room for improvement: for example, poor nutrition and inadequate housing are known to affect the health and growth of the mother and thus her capacity to bear healthy children; stress or malnutrition during pregnancy influences the baby at the time and subsequently; extreme parental rejection may lead to 'deprivation dwarfism'; and chronic malnutrition in early childhood has been linked to mental retardation.

Intellectual development

Now it is no longer held that functional intelligence is entirely innate. Like physical growth, it needs appropriate nourishment for its development. Moreover, 'man has by no means reached the limits of his mental powers; there is immense room for improvement at the lower end of the scale, and the possibility of more effective "techniques" at the top end' (Vernon, 1972).

As for translating this comparatively new knowledge into practice, there has as yet been little general or systematic attempt to do so. The exact contributions made respectively by genetic and environmental factors are still under debate; as is the question of whether 'thinking' needs to be taught as a separate skill (de Bono, 1972). Nor is there agreement on the optimal time, the most effective methods or the respective roles of home and school in fostering intellectual growth.

Educational development

That there is much room for improvement in this area is unanimously accepted. Evidence showing that this is indeed so is reliable and plentiful. There is less agreement on the causes of scholastic shortcomings or on the most appropriate methods for helping children to overcome them. Some concepts continue to be controversial, such as under-achievement, educational subnormality and dyslexia; there is also disagreement about basic teaching methods for, say, reading; about the effectiveness of different remedial treatments; about the merits of segregating handicapped children; and about many other basic educational issues, such as streaming, examinations and corporal punishment.

Extreme solutions, such as free schools, schools without walls, making education optional at an earlier age than at present, or abolishing compulsion altogether, have so far met with limited support.

In the United States the most consistent attempts to provide alternatives within the state school system are the voucher experiments, already under way in a few areas. By channelling public money for education through the parents in the form of vouchers, it is hoped to introduce a much more diverse range of options (Coons and Sugarman, 1978). While a similar scheme is unlikely to be introduced in this country, there is scope within the system for providing real choices. These could be initiated by existing schools, or groups of teachers, or parents or older students. They would offer a range of small-scale experiments whose importance, however, might well be out of all proportion to their size as a testing ground for real alternatives to formal schooling, especially at the secondary level. In that way they would come to fill the innovative role which progressive independent schools used to perform in the past.

Emotional and social development

These aspects of growth are the least explored and the results of available studies are usually neither clear-cut nor conclusive. This is clearly documented in a review of the short- and long-term effects of 'maternal deprivation' (Rutter, 1972 and 1979).

It had been thought that rising standards of health and material prosperity would reduce the incidence of backwardness, maladjustment and delinquency. There is evidence to suggest that to some extent, this has already happened. For example, children whose parents have been re-housed do better at school than those who remain in over-crowded conditions; and the delinquency rate is higher in slum areas than on well-established housing estates.

Yet it has become evident that the problems of emotional, social and educational malfunctioning will not be solved by improvements in health and in standards of living alone; these make satisfactory family and community life more likely but do not ensure it. Few would deny that there is much room for improvement at a time when vandalism, violence, drugs and crime are causing widespread concern.

Yet there has been no attempt to raise the general level of emotional and social resilience; indeed considerable resistance and suspicion surround even the discussion of this possibility, fears being voiced of brain-washing, social engineering and political manipulation. Instead, we must face the fact that these processes have been at work from time immemorial. Our various prejudices – be they about race, colour, class, sex or religion – are witness to that. The cost of refusing or neglecting to tackle directly the fostering of social and emotional maturity and resilience has been and continues to be very high in terms of human fulfilment and effectiveness.

MEANS OF BRINGING ABOUT IMPROVEMENT

At present, very considerable resources are being devoted to the treatment or containment of the disturbed, backward or delinquent; and when two out of every three known burglars are under twenty-one years old, there is clamour that more ought to be done. Yet neither child guidance clinics nor schools for the maladjusted have as yet produced convincing evidence of long-term success. Similarly, the success or failure rate of approved schools (measured in terms of recidivism) did not suggest that their style of treatment had found the answer.

It is evident that as yet we know little about why one child becomes delinquent when another in apparently similar circumstances does not; more is known about the general social and emotional conditions in which anti-social behaviour is likely to arise, and it is realised that its roots often go back into childhood (Robins, 1966; West, 1969; West and Farrington, 1974).

In the past twenty-five years many of the physical illnesses of childhood have been virtually eliminated. Tuberculosis of bones, joints, glands, digestive tract and meninges have almost disappeared with the control of bovine tuberculosis and the sterilization of milk supplies. Diphtheria and poliomyelitis have yielded to immunization of the child against the infecting organism. These victories, and a host of others, have been made possible because painstaking research has revealed eradicable causes of these diseases.

But a less encouraging picture is presented when we assess accomplishments in the field of mental and social health of the child. Here, there are to be heard no jubilant strains of victory; indeed, no unbiased observer can fail to be impressed with the poverty of achievement. Research in the mental, behavioural and social sciences has hitherto attracted too few of our best brains and attracted far too little financial encouragement (Cohen, 1965).

Thus, our state of knowledge in these areas is akin to that which prevailed in the health field some forty years ago. Might not the strategy, so conspicuously successful in that area, be appropriate also to other aspects of development? This is the fifth basic concept propounded in this book. Spectacular progress began to be made when it was accepted that 'the treatment of established disease is a most inefficient way of ensuring that we survive in good health... it is good preventive medicine and improved hygiene that does so, through the unostentatious departments of public health' (Malleson, 1973).

By providing maternity and child welfare clinics, by ensuring that children and pregnant mothers received the care and nourishment needed for proper growth, a virtual revolution was brought about within a generation. For example, fifty years ago, some 80 per cent of children in London's East End schools had signs of rickets and hence remained stunted in stature. Now the disease has almost been eliminated.

Just as it proved possible to vaccinate and inoculate successfully against whooping cough or poliomyelitis without necessarily understanding why a particular child was more liable to contract the disease or how to cure it, so there is now an understanding of the broad preventive measures likely to raise the general level of children's intellectual, educational, social and emotional development.

The developmental sciences offer evidence in, as yet, rather broad terms, which enables the environmental circumstances favouring or disfavouring the full development of human genetic potential to be, in an actuarial sense, prescribed. One of society's problems is to learn how to use this knowledge, particularly since evidence points to the crucial importance of long-term domestic environments over which, unlike schools, society exercises little control (Clarke and Clarke, 1972).

Even before birth the infant is a responsive and responding creature. For example, during the latter part of pregnancy the foetus can see and hear: a soft red light or certain kinds of sound cause it to turn slowly, while a bright light and certain noises can startle the unborn child. Thus the growing understanding of the earliest stages of human development indicates how early 'early' is. Even the intra-uterine environment and the first few days and weeks of life are significant for the infant's future development. It is then that the mother and child begin to interact and influence one another.

Studies have been carried out on the 'bonding' of mother and and infant by encouraging body contact, nursing and care straight after delivery and in the following few days, and assessing long-term results. Findings about the outcome vary; although such early contact is not essential for healthy mothering it has been found to be valuable, sometimes showing measurable results for a considerable time (Herbert et al., 1982; Klaus and Kennell, 1982; Goldberg, 1983).

Though the new-born child can adapt to widely different environments, to begin with he has a quite limited range of innate behavioural mechanisms. In consequence, the baby is entirely dependent upon the environment and 'the building block of nearly all human societies is the nuclear family' (Wilson, 1975). Thus for the purpose of social action and policy, the environment, and the family in particular, is of overriding importance. Indeed, all available evidence confirms that, from a practical viewpoint, the most important element in shaping behaviour and development is the environment in general and more specifically other human beings (White et al., 1979).

Hence prevention – and where need be intervention – must start long before a child's birth and continue throughout its childhood. Also, it is likely to be most effective and least costly – in terms of personnel, time and techniques – not merely during the earliest years but the earliest weeks and months of life; and also most effective if a start is made with today's children – the parents of tomorrow. On this argument, too, rests the case for preparing and then supporting parents who undertake the vital task of child-rearing – vital not only for their own children but also for society's future well-being.

2. The Needs of Children and How They Are Met

It used to be thought that developmental needs come into play in a hierarchical sequence, the most basic being those necessary for sheer survival (such as the need for food and water); and that only when these have been satisfactorily met do the higher needs emerge (such as the need for a loving relationship). Now it is held that all human needs are inter-related and inter-dependent in a subtle, complex and continuous way. For example, an unhappy baby may reject food and, even if he takes it, he may fail to thrive; or a child may fight sleep for fear that his mother or father may leave home.

It was also believed that the infant's attachment to his mother arose from her providing him with nourishment. Evidence has shown that this 'cupboard love' theory is not justified either, not even among monkeys. Similarly, emotion and learning were considered to be separate, distinct aspects of development; indeed this view is still widely held, particularly in relation to older children.

In fact learning (in the widest sense of the word) and emotion, the cognitive and affective aspects of development, intellect and feelings, are so closely interwoven and from so early an age as to be almost indivisible. Given inborn potential for development; given the impetus of maturation; and given environmental opportunities of an appropriate kind and at the appropriate time – what can still be missing is the willingness or motivation to learn and make progress. The essential driving force of the will to learn has its roots in the quality of relationships available to the child right from the beginning of life.

While parental love, and mothering in particular, has always been held to be important for children, social scientists continue to fight shy of the concept of 'mother-love', regarding it as unmeasurable, sentimental or both. Partly in consequence, practitioners have also undervalued it, if not in their daily attitudes to children and their families, then certainly in their staff training procedures. In 1951 a milestone was reached when Bowlby put forward the view – argued much earlier by Pestalozzi, Froebel and then Spitz – that 'mother-love in infancy and childhood is as important for mental health as are vitamins and proteins for physical health'. Now widely accepted by 'tender-minded' theorists and practitioners, its vagueness continues to arouse unease, even hostility, among the 'tough-minded'; so much so, that the word 'love' either appears in quotation marks or other terms, such as 'warmth' or 'attachment', are substituted.

Admittedly 'love' is not readily defined in scientific terms nor easily measurable. However, the elements which go to make up good parental care can be readily defined and many of the aspects of parent-child interaction can be assessed and evaluated. Much is now known about the ways in which the quality of family relationships affect children's development; and even more is known about the probable consequences when they are unsatisfactory or completely absent.

The position taken here is that even at its lowest the term 'maternal love' is a convenient shorthand; and, within the context of what follows, the role it plays in meeting children's developmental needs will become readily apparent. Since physical ones are not only more clearly understood but also more easily and now more generally met, the emphasis will be on psycho-social needs. These have been enumerated in lists, varying in length from as few as two to as many as sixty.

For practical purposes, a four-fold classification seems sufficient: the need for love and security; for new experiences; for praise and recognition; and for responsibility. These needs have to be met from the very beginning of life and continue to require fulfilment – to a greater or lesser extent – throughout adulthood. Of course, their relative importance changes during the different developmental stages as do the ways in which they are met.

THE NEED FOR LOVE AND SECURITY

The need for love

This need is met by the child experiencing from birth onwards a stable, continuous, dependable and loving relationship with his parents (or permanent parent-substitutes), who themselves enjoy a rewarding relationship with one another. Through this relationship – first with his mother, then his father and gradually an ever-widening circle of other people – the child comes to a realisation of personal identity and worthwhileness. It forms the basis of all later relationships, not only with the family, but with friends, colleagues and eventually his own family. On it depend the healthy development of the personality, the ability to respond to affection and, in time, to become a loving, caring parent.

The basic and all-pervasive feature of parental love is that the child is valued unconditionally and for his own sake, irrespective of his sex, appearance, abilities or personality; that this love is given without expectation of or demand for gratitude; and that the constraints imposed upon parental freedom of movement, upon time and upon finance are accepted without resentment or reproach. (Occasionally begrudging these constraints is, of course, different from a permanent sense of resentment.) Parents communicate this unconditional affection through all their relations with him: from physical care and handling to responding to his first smile and sounds; from protecting him from, and then gradually initiating him into, the social world; and from restraining to eventually punishing him for going beyond the limits they have set for acceptable behaviour.

The greatest impact of such love is on the self. Approval and acceptance by others are essential for the development of self-approval and self-acceptance. Whether a child will develop a constructive or destructive attitude, first to himself and then to other people, depends in the first place on his parents' attitude to him. During the earliest months of infancy and biological helplessness, the mother acts as insulator and filter, protecting the baby from the impact of his new environment. For example, a loud noise startles a baby far less, or a mild digestive upset will be endured more easily, when he is in his mother's or father's arms. Throughout the early years, close physical contact continues to be protectively reassuring, as well as an expression of parental affection. This is probably why, during the war, children who remained with their parents during bombing attacks coped better with anxiety than those who were evacuated to safer areas.

During this time, few demands are made on the infant and all his wants are met. It is he who at this early stage provides both the impetus and directive for maternal behaviour: she responds not only because of her concern for him but also for her own comfort, as his crying is painful to her. Following this period of total egocentricity the initiative passes to the mother: the baby is expected to begin to give up instant gratification, to accept postponement and to respond to the requirements of others; this sets him on the way – slowly and often painfully – to becoming integrated into a wider social world. From now on the relationship becomes and continues to be a reciprocal one.

Though able to respond to sights and sounds within the first forty-eight hours of life, the first truly social step is the infant's smile responding to a smiling face. This happens in about the second month of life; only several months later does he become able to identify and differentiate his mother's face from that of others. This is an important milestone: it marks the emergence of his awareness of his mother as a separate person, 'outside himself' as it were, and thus the beginning of his identity or self-concept; it also marks the growth of his first and vital emotional attachment or bond. To reach this stage, he has had to accomplish a vast amount of learning so as to be able to distinguish between a host of sensory impressions.

From this first reciprocal love relationship flow three further consequences of vital importance to development: first, the baby enjoys the mother's presence, even if he can only hear her moving about, and he becomes concerned when she disappears. Secondly, the loving mother who watches and encourages each step forward is likely to accelerate progress by her anticipatory interest and delight in the earliest signs; these 'reward' the baby for his efforts and spur him on to continue making them. Hence he may learn to walk and talk earlier than a child whose mother has not the time or inclination for such close involvement in his progress. Conversely, she conveys disappointment and disapproval of behaviour which she wishes to discourage.

The third consequence is that the child is enabled through mutually rewarding relationships, first with his mother and then with others who become significant to him, to learn self-control and to acquire moral values. This he accomplishes by imitation or 'modelling'. Mothering mediates between the child's inner subjective and the outside 'real' world; it recognises and establishes his personal identity and individuality; and her loving care is unique in the sense that it is adapted to his very special, individual needs which are recognised as being different from those of any other child.

Such love is extremely difficult to replace and hence it makes the child vulnerable when it is lost to him, temporarily or permanently. In most cases 'The best that community care can offer is impartiality – to be fair to every child in its care. But a developing personality needs more than that: it needs to know that to someone it matters more than other children; that someone will go to unreasonable lengths... for its sake' (Newson, 1972).

The need for security

First and foremost, this need is met by giving the child the security of stable family relationships where attitudes and behaviour are consistent and dependable; the security of a familiar place; and the security of a known routine. All these make for continuity and predictability in a world in which the child has to meet and come to terms with so much that is new and changing.

Because he is so small and so ignorant, much that is later taken for granted is seen as threatening; for example, such simple things as the water running out of the bath. Similarly, the unpredictability of objects can be frightening, such as glass breaking when dropped. Perhaps most of all, the nature and strength of his own feelings threaten his security from time to time. If the whole framework of his life is secure, it provides him with the needed reassurance to venture out, knowing that he can again return to its comforting safety.

It is the quality of family relationships which is of basic importance to the child's psychological development. This applies not only to the mother's and father's relations with him, but also to those between the parents themselves, as well as to the child's with his siblings and other close relatives. Parental expectation and discipline which are consistent – whether tending to be strict or lenient – enhance his sense of security, providing a dependable predictable framework. So does a familiar place, as is clearly shown by the contrast between a young child's usual behaviour in his own home and in a strange place. Keeping close to his mother or a familiar person, refusing to speak or eat, are all signs of insecurity. A familiar object gives reassurance, as witnessed by a cherished possession – often something cuddly such as a rag doll or blanket – from which he will not be parted at bedtime or in a stressful situation.

The extent to which a known routine helps the growing child is shown by his insistence that certain everyday events are followed in exactly the same manner and sequence; bedtime rituals and the way stories must be told in the self-same words are just two examples. Parents are in a unique position to know about the particular objects, rituals and situations which foster a particular child's sense of security. By allowing them expression (and time where need be), his right to individuality and to a measure of self-determination is acknowledged, which contributes towards building up his feeling of worth.

There are two further aspects to allowing him the right to certain idiosyncrasies within the home: first, the fact that the child can revert to more immature behaviour becomes a valuable safety valve in the face of the constant and increasing demands on him for greater maturity and control; and secondly, he begins to learn that different standards of behaviour are permitted within the privacy of his family, which will help him later to understand and cope with this fact in relation to school and other social settings.

The need for security is closely related to the standards of behaviour being set by the parents. Knowing what is expected of him and, as soon as he can understand, the reasons why, makes growing up a less difficult business. Inevitably the child will transgress, will be disobedient – partly because he needs to test the consequences of doing so, partly because he is liable to forget rules – but knowing the limits of what is permitted provides the reassurance of both reasonableness and predictability. In contrast, when the same behaviour gives rise to widely different reactions, with the same parent at different times or in either parent, then the child's concept of acceptable conduct becomes linked to individual whim rather than to general principles.

Lastly, but perhaps most important, stable family life also provides the child with a sense of personal continuity, of having a past as well as a future. By relating to him events of his early life, backed up by photos and other evidence, and by looking ahead to likely developments in his life, he acquires a coherent self-image which is essential for a well-adjusted personality. Children love hearing stories about their own doings. These together with comments made casually in conversation about other members of the family all serve to accumulate a store of memories which put his own life into long-term perspective. 'When you were younger' and 'when you are older' are phrases which may well at times irritate children by the very frequency with which they are used; yet they contribute to building up a mental concept of his continuing self within the larger family context. It is through human ties that personal identity comes to be established.

Teacher–pupil relations

Since the relationships available to the child are of paramount importance, one would expect the teacher to become one of the most influential adults in the child's expanding world – after all he stands *in loco parentis* during a large part of the day; so much so, that a deprived child will often address a teacher to whom he becomes attached as 'mummy'.

In a review of some fifty studies, carried out in recent years, on the way in which teachers' behaviour affects the achievements of their pupils, two aspects were consistently found to be important: teacher enthusiasm and warmth (Rosenshine, 1971). These not only elicit greater response from each individual but they also create for the whole class a climate of involvement reflected in the attitudes of pupils to each other, to the teacher and to learning.

Disapproval and discipline

Once a child has learned through a loving mother's response to him that he is valued and cherished, this satisfying experience is 'ever afterwards craved and so constitutes a powerful driving force of human nature' (Moore, T. V., 1948).

Disapproval is felt as a temporary withdrawal of affection and is sensed long before the child can understand speech or talk himself. Even later, speech is not necessary: facial expressions – a frown, a smile or even a raised eyebrow – can at times be more eloquent and effective than words. Indeed, such non-verbal communication remains a potent means of conveying displeasure way beyond childhood. Thus if his mother is displeased with him, the child becomes anxious.

Later the disapproval of others, who are emotionally significant to the child, will also induce anxiety. In this way, the loving relationships formed in early infancy provide the most effective and basic motivation for a child to respond increasingly to adult expectations. Throughout his childhood, he will adapt to parental training, demands and guidance because he wants to retain their love; transgression means the interruption of this valued relationship, because feeling disapproved of is painful to his self-image and because anxiety is such a disturbing emotion that he endeavours to avoid behaviour likely to arouse it.

The fact that during adolescence many youngsters rebel against parental standards and seek to find their own way of solving problems in no way changes the need for parents to make clear what they regard as desirable or acceptable standards. The more loving and warmer the home, the easier it is for the child to discriminate between a continuing basic affection and what feels like its temporary loss (i.e., disapproval), because the signs or cues are quite distinct; this helps him to understand what is expected of him and facilitates his response. Inconsistent, erratic parental handling makes this more difficult since the cues will be contradictory and hence confusing. The situation is most difficult for the child who is rejected or being brought up in the more impersonal atmosphere of a children's home, since the cues will be blurred, if they exist at all; disapproval only confirms his feeling of being unloved. When he has no permanent parent figures, he has no hope of gaining or regaining their affection.

It is through a caring adult then that the child learns to care. To begin with, neither words nor actions are inherently right or wrong – it is the response they evoke which teaches him how they are regarded. It is not only consistency of response but also whether the adult himself provides a consistent model for the child, which will influence how readily he comes to understand what is expected of him. Since parents provide not only the first but also the most intimately observed models, their standards, values and disciplinary approach lay the basis for the child's eventual conduct; in particular, whether it becomes inner- or outer-directed.

In common usage, the term 'discipline' has become practically synonymous with punishment, and often has overtones of severity. Perhaps because of this, 'methods of child rearing' is a preferable term, though, in fact, the original definition of discipline is equally neutral, namely training which develops self-control and the capacity to cooperate. The more child rearing methods are based on reasoning and discussion, the more readily understanding develops of parental standards and expectations. This lays the basis for moral insight as a guide to behaviour rather than 'blind obedience' induced by either fear of punishment (whether physical or verbal lashings) or by the 'emotional blackmail' of withholding affection.

When behaviour is inner-directed, the child comes to feel shame and guilt when he is doing something which he knows his parents would disapprove of. To begin with, anxiety about parental displeasure and, later on, understanding of parental precepts induce him to adopt socially and morally acceptable behaviour by exercising self-control. In this way he eventually develops a 'conscience' through anticipating and internalising likely parental (and then increasingly other people's) expectations and reactions so that he will behave in an increasingly mature and self-directed manner, independent of the parents' physical presence.

Consistent and reasonable expectations which are appropriate to the child's age and level of understanding; punishments which are similarly consistent and logically related to the 'offence' (from having to forgo a treat to having to make restitution; and from being scolded to being temporarily isolated because of anti-social behaviour); and an open and 'democratic' family climate in which explanations are readily given; all these are conducive to emphasising the value of internal controls.

In contrast, outer-directed behaviour operates largely on an *ad hoc* basis, where 'love-orientated' methods of discipline cannot come into play, either because there is no continuing, warm relationship or because there is no consistent and appropriate pattern of parental expectation. Outer-directed behaviour relies heavily on rewards and punishment; is orientated towards the present; and adapted to the standards and expectations of a particular person or situation at a particular time.

Autocratic discipline, which is imposed from outside rather than accepted through identification with a loved person, has to rely more on punishment, fear and external control; it is these which come to regulate behaviour and ensure conformity. To evade detection and beat the system then become a challenge to the child.

THE NEED FOR NEW EXPERIENCES

New experiences are a prerequisite for mental growth as essential to the mind's development as food is for the body's. From birth onwards, tasks appropriate to each particular stage of growth are presented to the child, and their mastery provides in turn the stepping stone towards more difficult achievements: for example, from having learned to grasp and hold an object, he proceeds to learn to feed himself. If denied the opportunity of new experiences, no learning can take place. For example, in a non-speaking environment, the child will not acquire speech even though his hearing and speech organs are quite normal.

The small child has a strong urge to explore, and everything that goes on around him becomes an absorbing new experience as soon as he is able to perceive it; so is every one of his earliest accomplishments, be it the ability to move his limbs at will or to examine the texture, taste and shape of materials and objects. Similarly, learning to crawl, walk, run and climb are new experiences in themselves, in addition to opening up an increasingly wider world for first-hand exploration. Later still, the challenge will be the mastery of reading, riding a bicycle or climbing a mountain. All these, and many more, provide new fields to be conquered, making life for the normal active child a series of rewarding adventures.

Once interest in novelty appears, then it becomes increasingly important as a source of motivation for further exploration and thus for learning. In Piaget's words, 'the more an infant has seen and heard, the more he wants to see and hear'. At the same time, there can be too much or too little stimulation or 'input'; the former gives rise to withdrawal and fear, the latter to boredom and apathy. It is one of the skills of child-rearing to be able to judge accurately the optimal level which will foster the cognitive development of a particular child at any particular stage of his growth.

New experiences enable the child to learn one of the most important, because basic, lessons of early life: learning how to learn; and learning that mastery brings joy and a sense of achievement. This is demonstrated by the exultant cry of 'I can do it myself', which also illustrates the link between emotion and learning, between cognitive and affective experiences. Competence brings its own reward while the mother's or other adults' pleasure in the child's newly acquired skill further reinforces his willingness to seek new fields to conquer.

In contrast, the child whose exploratory activities are disapproved of, discouraged or punished – whether this is because they disorganise a tidy, smooth-running, adult-centred household, or because the potential hazards worry an anxious mother, or because in over-crowded conditions a harassed, over-burdened mother cannot provide either the time or space – such a child will develop quite another attitude to learning: its likely features will be passivity, fearfulness, frustration or irritability, and there will be little joy or satisfaction.

In this way, educability – a child's responsiveness to all the growth tasks to which education, in the very widest sense of the term, exposes him – depends not only on his inborn capacity, but on environmental opportunity and encouragement. The emotional and cultural climate of the home, as well as parental involvement and aspirations, can foster, limit or even impair intellectual growth. Potentialities for learning may be developed to the full, be disorganised or remain unrealised according to the nature of the child's environment.

Just as an appropriate diet is essential for normal physical growth, so it is for mental development. The most vital ingredients of this diet are play and language. Through them, the child explores the world and learns to cope with it; this is as true for the objective outside world of reality as it is for the subjective internal world of thoughts and feelings. Thus too are motor skills, perception and concepts developed.

The functions of play

The phrase 'he is only playing' is still far too often heard, implying that play is only slightly superior to doing nothing at all. In fact, it is an intensely absorbing experience and even more important to the child than work is to the adult. Hence it ought to be treated with similar respect. It fulfils a number of different though related functions, and takes many forms.

Perhaps the earliest play occurs at the breast with the baby's exploratory touching of the mother. If breast-fed babies thrive better – as is believed by many – it may be not only for nutritional reasons but also because, in addition to body contact, it provides the first mutually enjoyable play opportunity. Possibly too

an appreciation of the value of play begins at this stage and not simply later when the toddler is fitting blocks into holes. The middle class mother encourages the latter but may find it difficult to tolerate the time-wasting involved in the former. The peasant mother, and this includes some immigrant mothers, may be particularly responsive to the former, but cannot see the importance of a toddler's exploratory activities unless she is taught the why and how of play (Kitzinger, 1973).

Play also enables the baby to acquire control over his body. Through moving his limbs and exercising his muscles, coordination develops and in playing he sets himself increasingly difficult tasks; for example, from crawling to walking and running; and from jumping to hopping on one foot, and eventually to playing complex games.

Next, children play with sounds, words and objects in a very similar way, partly to practise newly developing skills, partly to acquire new knowledge and partly for the sheer joy of it. The babbling baby who tries to imitate the sounds his mother makes has his counterpart in the older child who chants difficult words which intrigue him; while the chanting of nonsense rhymes and jingles is fun, as well as giving a sense of power over words. Playing with materials such as sand and water, he learns about their different properties, just as he does when accidentally dropping a saucepan or jam jar on a hard floor.

For creative play, both words and objects are used. Pounding clay, smearing paint, erecting a brick structure, taking an old clock to pieces, playing a musical instrument or writing a poem, all these provide both a means for self-expression and for learning about and remaking the world as he experiences it. These activities also help to lay the cornerstone of his feelings about himself in relation to that world; while the foundation for later imaginative and artistic pursuits and appreciation is laid through music, movement and nursery rhymes.

There is yet another aspect of play. It provides not only an outlet for feelings but a means of coping with them. For example, the angry child has made a step forward when he kicks his teddy bear or a ball instead of the baby or the furniture; the next step is the child telling the teddy that it is naughty to kick and that he must learn more sensible means of containing his anger; when much later the child himself is able not only to control but to use his anger constructively – be this through hammering nails into wood to make a toy or by writing an essay attacking unduly repressive ways of disciplining children – then he is well on the way to maturity.

Two further aspects of play deserve mentioning, namely role-playing and make-believe. The former enables a child both to 'practise' his future identity as an adult, parent and worker; and to feel himself in imagination into the parts played by others, be it his mother, his teacher, the milkman or an astronaut. By learning to put himself 'into their shoes' he will become more adept later at cooperating with others. (Incidentally, it can be a salutary experience to realise through watching a child's expression and voice how he perceives the adults around him.)

One reason why boys show a higher incidence of emotional difficulties, not only in this country but in all developed countries which publish statistics, may be because it is less easy for them to observe, identify with and practise role-appropriate behaviour. The mother's home-making work is much more 'visible' to the young child than the father's job; this is true too for the early school years when boys are usually taught by women.

Make-believe games allow the child to anticipate through the medium of fantasy impending, and possibly frightening, experiences, such as having to go into hospital. He is enabled to assimilate new experiences by re-living them, such as after a visit to the zoo, when he will pretend to be each of the various animals he has seen. Perhaps most important of all, he can find temporary relief and refuge from being small, inexperienced and without any real power, by creating in his imaginative play a world where he is king, where his deepest wishes are fulfilled, and where it is he who makes and breaks the rules. In short, make-believe assists the child in working through and coming to terms with the frustrations and conflicts which are almost inseparable from growing up in a complex and fast-changing society.

Last, though by no means least, play is enjoyable not only for the child but also the adult. Partly because of the somewhat belittling attitude towards play referred to earlier and partly just because they enjoy it, some parents tend to feel that it must take very much second place to all the other tasks of home-making and family life, from shopping and cooking, to gardening and servicing the car. Yet if play is to provide the wide range of opportunities for learning, which it potentially can do, then adult involvement is essential.

Choosing toys, materials and equipment which are appropriate to the child's age and level of maturity requires care and understanding. Decisions need to be made not only as to quantity but also regarding the balance between 'raw' (i.e., clay or paints), constructional (i.e., bricks or Lego) and 'finished' (i.e., dolls or trains) materials.

Similarly, the balance between completely 'free' play, which is entirely of the child's own choosing and under his sole direction, and 'guided' activities, where the parent or teacher suggests, participates, contributes or even teaches and corrects, is an important matter. Moreover, for some children, the right atmosphere needs to be created for dramatic and spontaneous play; yet it may be inhibiting if the guiding adult injects or imposes the logic of objective reality or the pattern of adult imagination.

In summary, play can be seen to meet the need for new experiences in two major ways: by enabling the child to learn about the world he lives in; and by providing a means for learning about and resolving complex and often conflicting emotions, i.e., by fantasy being allowed to over-ride reality and logic. Thus a synthesis is brought about between the inner and outer world, between rational and non-rational processes, new understanding being absorbed through the child's individual prior store of ideas, images, feelings, wishes and conflicts.

The functions of language

The child who asked, 'How do I know what I think till I hear what I say?', neatly summarised the central role of language for intellectual functioning; indeed, thought itself has been defined as 'internalised speech'. The young child uses monologue a good deal, in a kind of running commentary on what he is doing. Whether this reflects his egocentricity at this stage (as Piaget suggests) or whether it is a sort of self-directive communication (as Vygotsky maintains) remains to be established as do many other aspects of speech.

Once a detailed understanding is achieved of how language is acquired, then substantial progress can be made with programmes designed to foster its growth. There is no doubt that language is basic to an effective cognitive life, because it makes rational thought possible. 'All of man's unique social behaviour pivots on his use of language' (Wilson, 1975).

Language development follows a regular sequential pattern, from babbling to short words and finally to sentences, which will increase in length and complexity. The child who is 'bathed in language' – whose mother talks while she plays with and does things for him, who tells him nursery rhymes, stories, sings and converses – such a child will be attuned to sounds from an early age. In turn, the first sounds he himself makes, which vaguely resemble real words, will be greeted with such pleasure by parents aware of the importance of early vocalising, that he is likely to repeat them more often until he does in fact connect the word with its object.

Being able to name things extends the child's power over his environment – he can identify and demand things instead of having to rely on his mother's guesswork of what he might be wanting. Vocalising also seems to bring its own reward; how else can one explain that babbling continues when the child does not want to communicate with anyone nor has an interested audience? Playing with words at an older age may well be a counterpart of this early activity.

Once the child has acquired some language and understands that words refer to things, child-rearing becomes easier. Communication is improved and speech also provides the child with increasing control over himself as well as his environment. For example, the word 'no' makes it possible for him to reach out to touch something hot and then to control the impulse himself by the incantation of the parental prohibition, which had checked him on previous occasions.

Thus language plays a part not only in learning self-control but in the formation of conscience. Also, with increasing age the child comes to appreciate that verbal aggression is socially more acceptable than its physical expression and that it can be equally effective, even if not quite as immediately satisfying. Similarly, through words he begins to form concepts and to generalise; for example, he will learn to distinguish between cats and dogs, and to comprehend that both are animals. Gradually, with increasing linguistic facility, the higher mental processes of reasoning and judgement will begin to develop.

Though there are wide individual variations among children, eight-year-olds have on average acquired 50 per cent of the vocabulary they will have at the age of eighteen. Generally speaking, girls are ahead of boys in language development – until the age of eight years, if not later – whether the yardsticks used for assessment are speech sounds, articulation, vocabulary or sentence structure.

Also, at every age, children from middle class homes are ahead of those in working class homes. It is not simply a question of the latter reaching the same level but at a somewhat later age; rather, the whole mode of language differs, from a smaller vocabulary to the use of shorter, simpler and often incomplete sentences; also, subordinate clauses, adjectives and adverbs are employed less imaginatively and frequently. Language, furthermore, shapes both thought and behaviour.

The most systematic study of children's thinking has been made by Piaget who demonstrated that cognitive development passes through stages of increasing complexity, the sequence of which is not readily altered. The 'sensory-motor' period is the first and lasts about two years. At this stage, the infant's knowledge of the world depends on his bodily interaction with and his actual handling of objects.

Next comes the period of 'pre-operational thought' which lasts until about seven years. During it, the child is beginning to think symbolically, with speech playing an increasing part. For example, when he pretends to be driving a car, while sitting in a cardboard box, he symbolises his past experience and relates it to the present. These two stages are dominated by his immediate perception, and thinking is on what Piaget calls the 'intuitive level'.

The third stage, which lasts until about eleven years, he calls the period of 'concrete operations' and the final one, which is accomplished by about fifteen years, the period of 'formal operations'. During the former, most of the child's thinking is still based on concrete objects or specific situations; he cannot as yet transfer what he has learned in one physical context to another. For example, the concept of 'conservation' of volume requires the understanding that certain properties (in this case the volume) of objects remain constant even when other properties (e.g., the shape) are changed. Most eight-year-olds know that pouring water from a tall thin container into a short broad one does not change the amount of water; but only by about eleven years will there be the ability to comprehend that the volume of the two containers is also the same. In other words, the capacity for hypothetico-deductive reasoning is reached in the period of 'formal operations'. It is only then that abstract thinking becomes possible.

By his work, Piaget has shown that children's thinking is qualitatively different from adult thought; however, his studies are not concerned with age-related norms and considerable variability has in fact been found among children. Also, he argues that there is constant interaction between emotions and intellect so that during stress a child will regress to an earlier level of thinking. Presumably, too, emotional difficulties may prevent a child from ever reaching a higher level of logical functioning, so that unresolved emotional conflict at one level of development will hinder thinking at the next level.

Here then is one link between language, thought and behaviour. Others are even more important because more generalised and pervasive. The use of simpler, less individualised language – more habitual among working class homes – is likely to mean that small or subtle differences between objects, people and situations are ignored; also, the nuances of wishes and feeling will be more difficult to convey with more restricted speech. In consequence, children will grow up less sensitive to their own emotions and those of others; less able to distinguish the finer shades of meanings; and in their thinking they may well remain at the 'concrete' level, never passing to the level of 'formal operations'.

In summary, language helps children to learn to reason, to think and to understand the world around them; speech facilitates the making of relationships, both with adults and with contemporaries; and verbal communication is and remains a vital means of coping and coming to terms with life. Eventually, the child's response to school and the progress he is able to make will depend in no small measure on his ability to express himself, and on his mastery and enjoyment of the spoken word.

Social class differences

Why should speech and thought processes of children from working class homes tend to be more limited in range, subtlety and sensitivity? Two main hypotheses have been put forward to account for this differential language development (Bernstein, 1961; Hess and Shipman, 1965; Newson, 1972). First, middle class children generally live in a verbally much richer environment where they are encouraged to listen and respond to increasingly more mature speech patterns; where stories, nursery rhymes and word games are an important part of daily routine; and where conversation is freely engaged in, for example at meal times, during shopping and at bed-time, rather than being regarded as time-wasting chatter.

Secondly, working class and middle class homes tend to differ in their style of child rearing, the former favouring an 'authoritarian' and the latter a more 'democratic' form of discipline. In democratic homes, the reasons for expected behaviour and for rules are explained, verbal means of control are preferred to physical, and the child's views and wishes are taken into account in decision making. So in addition to the greater inclination for verbal interchange, there is also a greater need for it in 'democratic' homes. This means that there are more frequent, prolonged and reciprocal interactions between parents and children. These foster two other aspects of behaviour: a readiness to approach new problems with an open mind and a sense of personal independence (Wall, 1973; Entwistle, 1978).

On the other hand, less conversation is needed in the 'authoritarian' home since mainly non-verbal means of prohibition and punishment are employed, and words are used more to threaten and enforce obedience rather than to make the child understand the rationale behind social behaviour. It may well be that cuffs and blows are resorted to more often by working class parents partly because they are less able to put their feelings into words. The use of actual physical violence in socially impoverished or disturbed homes is likely to produce poorly socialised children who will then carry the same behaviour into the next generation.

Thus these two different ways of upbringing – conveyed through language – generate a different family 'climate' which in turn shapes behaviour and personality. On going to school, the child is expected to adopt the language of mainly middle class teachers and to cope with a largely middle class curriculum. Whether this necessarily creates difficulties will be discussed later (Chapter 5, p. 101).

The teacher's role

Going to school is itself a major new experience, which opens up a larger and more impersonal world. Fortunate is the child who can be introduced gradually rather than having to adapt suddenly to spending the greater part of his day away from his mother, in unfamiliar surroundings with a strange adult for whose attention he has to compete with many strange contemporaries. In addition to this unaccustomed sharing, it may also be a new experience for him to have to compare himself with his peers.

Inevitably his previous attitudes to new experiences will be reflected in his response; his mother's attitude to 'losing' him as well as her views of education in general, and to his school in particular, will also affect his own expectations and adjustment. Since the regime of most infant schools is child-centred and 'discovery' orientated, at least during the first year, most children show little difficulty in coping with this major change in their lives, provided that their curiosity and exploratory activities have previously been fostered.

The child's progress will come to be powerfully affected by his teacher's attitudes, values and beliefs; some of these will be overt and deliberate; others may be implicit and incidental; still others may well be unconscious but just as powerful in influencing his learning (Pilling and Pringle, 1978). Wide interests, enthusiasm for things of the mind and receptiveness to new ideas – all these are infectious. Many a child has had new doors opened by, and chosen his life's work because of, an inspired teacher.

However, as he advances up the educational ladder, he is likely to find school becoming increasingly 'achievement' orientated, subject-centred and competitive. Indeed, the progressive ideas of primary education, with their stress on stimulating inquiry and discovery by pupils through largely self-chosen activities, have aroused considerable doubts, both among secondary schools and the public at large; yet there is no necessary incompatibility between these ideas and high standards of attainment.

> Schools can be genuinely concerned with gaiety and joy and individual growth and fulfilment, without sacrificing concern for intellectual discipline and development. They can be simultaneously child-centred and knowledge-centred. They can stress aesthetic and moral education without weakening the three R's (Silberman, 1970).

Perhaps the most important role of the teacher in opening up new worlds to the child is by being a bridge-builder. Four aspects will be singled out. The first concerns the relation between emotion and learning. Schools have for far too long over-emphasised the place of cognitive abilities and underestimated the importance of motivation. Instead, it needs to be recognised that the major determinant of educational success lies in bridging the two. To do so requires teachers to have an optimistic attitude; to accept that wanting to know and to seek evidence, and knowing how and where to find information, are more important and lasting than mere rote learning; to adopt teaching methods which maximise the strength and minimise the weakness of each pupil; and to devise a curriculum which is relevant to his interests and stage of development. Because neither interest nor stages are watertight entities, rigid boundaries between different subjects, and between nursery, primary, middle and secondary schools are inappropriate.

Next, the school should bridge the world of the child's home and the community at large. The teacher, by involving himself, as well as his pupils, in outward-looking activities, which include both the parents and the neighbourhood, will discover unsuspected resources of ingenuity and initiative. Current thinking on bringing parents into much closer relationship with their children's schooling and making the premises a focal point of neighbourhood life, to some extent also aims to foster greater parental and community involvement (Tizard et al., 1981). By providing a better understanding of the purpose of new methods of teaching and learning, parental interests may be enlisted; this in turn is likely to influence the children's attitudes and achievements. However, neither project work nor group teaching nor community use of premises is feasible in traditional classrooms; hence, these must become a thing of the past in primary and secondary schools alike.

Thirdly, the teacher is best placed to build bridges between education and the other professions most closely concerned with the development and well-being of children (Fitzherbert, 1977). In order to promote greater inter-disciplinary cooperation at the 'grass roots', people need to come together from different professional fields and from the statutory and voluntary services, in a variety of activities based on the school as a neighbourhood resource centre. Then education could be carried on 'against a relevant and recognisable background of human interaction and responsiveness rather than in an over-protected, over-regulated institution in danger of losing touch with its changing purposes' (Cooksey, 1972).

The fourth aspect of bridge-building relates to being an innovator. Perhaps the best teacher has always tried to be ahead of his time, recognising that education should be for tomorrow; it is stagnant if it prepares only for today and fossilised if appropriate mainly for yesterday's world. This is why society must be prepared to support and even encourage what Schon has called 'the vanguard role of the teacher' (5th Reith Lecture, 13 December 1970). This means openness and flexibility on the teacher's part: learning himself as he adopts the new methods and new techniques which educational technology has to offer; retaining what he finds valuable in traditional approaches; and discarding what fails to fulfil its promise in the new ways. Just as children become truly considerate only when shown consideration by their parents and teachers, so it is only the teacher whose own thinking is flexible who will succeed in imparting a receptive and adaptive attitude of mind.

By these various means, teachers will be able to preserve or to rekindle the curiosity and joy in learning shown by the young child which stand in such stark contrast to the frustrated boredom of not a few secondary school pupils (Banks and Finlayson, 1973; Wall, 1977).

THE NEED FOR PRAISE AND RECOGNITION

Because growing from a helpless baby into a self-reliant adult requires an enormous amount of emotional, social and intellectual learning and because it is inevitably beset by difficulties, conflicts and setbacks, a strong incentive is needed. This is provided by the pleasure shown at success and by the praise given to achievement by the adults who love the child and whom he in turn loves and wants to please. Encouragement and a reasonable level of expectation act as a spur to perseverance. Too little expectation leads the child to adopt too low a standard of effort and achievement; too high a level makes him feel that he cannot live up to what is required of him which produces discouragement and again diminished effort. An optimal level of expectation needs to be geared to each individual's capabilities at a given point in time and stage of growth, at a level where success is possible but not without effort.

Mistakes and failure should be regarded as an integral part of learning for which he is neither disapproved of nor scolded. Of course, this does not mean a child should never be reproved, be required to make restitution, or be punished; refusal to do something he is capable of doing, deliberate disobedience or destructiveness are quite different from mishaps, like breaking an ornament because of not yet being able to discriminate between breakable and unbreakable objects, or mistakes due to lack of knowledge, such as spelling errors. The child who is made to feel anxious because of his mistakes, often becomes more concerned about avoiding anxiety which is painful, than about analysing and profiting from the reasons for his failure. Also, he needs to feel that learning is unhurried and that successful accomplishment is largely a matter of time.

Teachers also play a key role – for better or worse – in meeting the need for praise and recognition: they are the only profession in close and continued contact with all children for at least eleven years; and from the age of five years at the latest, every child spends about half his waking life in school. This provides an unrivalled opportunity not only to establish a favourable attitude to learning in general and scholastic progress in particular; but also, where necessary, to improve or entirely rebuild the foundation for a child's self-esteem and hence his attitude to learning.

To accomplish this, a teacher has to act on the assumption that every pupil possesses an as yet unrealised potential for development; that an appropriate 'diet' can succeed in improving intellectual or emotional 'under-nourishment;' and that rather than accepting previous assessments or test results or even the parents' judgement of the child's abilities, the teacher should try to 'beat prediction'. even though he may not always succeed.

Such a positive and optimistic attitude communicates itself very readily. Even such minimal 'signals' as raised eyebrows, smiles, nods and encouraging 'hms' effectively influence (or 'reinforce') attitude and performance. After all, a child's self-concept is developed through the views others hold of him. If he is called slow, he feels stupid – his yardstick can only be that of the adults who matter to him. Even very bright children may think of themselves as failures if their ability remains unrecognised; the number of such 'able misfits', as I have called them, is by no means negligible – thousands pass through our schools each year (Pringle, 1970; Dowdall and Colangelo, 1982).

A child's attitude to himself and to learning will determine how effectively he learns, as much as, if not more than, his actual abilities. Recognition from his teacher and his peers assumes increasing importance with increasing age, the influence of the latter reaching a peak during adolescence. Eventually, a job well done becomes its own reward but that is a very mature stage, not usually reached before adolescence; and even the most mature adult responds, and indeed blossoms, when given – at least occasionally – some praise or other form of recognition by those whose views he values.

> If the school environment provides the individual with evidence of his adequacy over a number of years, especially in the first few years of school, supported by consistent success over the next four of five years, we believe that this provides a type of immunisation against mental illness for an indefinite period of time. Such an individual should be able to surmount crises and periods of great stress without suffering too much. His own sense of adequacy and his

personal and technical skills (some learned in school) should enable him to use realistic methods in surmounting these crisis situations (Bloom, 1974).

THE NEED FOR RESPONSIBILITY

This need is met by allowing the child to gain personal independence, to begin with through learning to look after himself in matters of his everyday care, such as feeding, dressing and washing himself. Because he is constantly modelling himself on his parents, he wants to imitate what they can do. Despite the difficulties and frustrations arising from his immaturity and lack of control, he demands the chance to struggle on; hence 'me do it' is the constant refrain of the two-year-old. This need is met too through having possessions, however small and inexpensive, over which the child is allowed to exercise absolute ownership.

As he grows older, increasing independence means permitting, indeed encouraging, increasing freedom – of physical movement; of taste in food, play and clothes; and, perhaps most important of all, of choice of friends, studies, hobbies, career and eventually marriage partner. Giving such independence does not mean withholding one's views, tastes and choices, or the reasons for them; nor does it mean opting out from participating and guiding the lives of children; nor, indeed, condoning everything they may do.

On the contrary, children need a framework of guidance, of limits – knowing what is expected or permitted and what the rules are – together with the reasons and whether these are in their interests or in the interests of others. This means that it is important to distinguish clearly between disapproval of their behaviour, on the one hand, and on the other rejection of the child himself; and that the only lasting and effective force for influencing their beliefs and behaviour is the model we ourselves provide: it is what we really are and how we behave which matters, not what we say or believe we are. By sharing our everyday lives, children learn about our values, standards, concerns and ambitions in a subtle yet pervasively influential way.

Young people also need

> experience in coping with egalitarian relationships with their immediate peers and contemporaries apart from the normal setting in which they are invariably subordinate to adults. Having learned in

association with parents, teachers and older kinsfolk to come to some kind of terms with authority and to adjust to externally imposed codes of behaviour, they need a period in which they relate to others as equals and so learn to stand on their own feet. Only in age-homogeneous peer groups can true equality be found and thus it is as members of such youth groups that vital steps towards ultimate autonomy and independence have to be made. So the college sorority, the street corner gang, the orthodox youth club, the students' union, the spontaneous sports team, the 'clique', personal friends, mates or pals fulfil an important social and psychological function which must necessarily to some extent make their members feel themselves distinct from other groups and generations. A great amount of emotion is usually invested in peer-group and friendship relationships at the adolescent stage. The group solidarity and companionship often generate a warmth and romanticism which give youth an almost transcendental glow and rapture never to be regained (Mays, 1974).

How can responsibility be given to the immature and to the irresponsible? There is no way out of the dilemma that unless it is granted, the child cannot learn how to exercise it. Like every other skill, it needs to be practised under adult guidance which then gradually diminishes during adolescence and adulthood. That it is worth taking the risks involved has been shown by the work of those who make this a central issue of their care for deprived, disturbed or delinquent young people.

Yet to some extent, family, school and society may be failing to provide sufficient and sufficiently graded training for responsibility and autonomy. It has been suggested

> That the road to maturity lies through the construction of four selves – social, sexual, vocational and philosophic . . . in these four areas adolescents are driven to make a series of responsible choices which – if they are real and stable ones – no human being can take for another; they are also matters where knowledge and information are essential to wise decisions; because so often the consequences of choice look so irrevocable, and the young feel themselves so inexperienced, the very need to choose may provoke acute anxiety or even panic (Wall, 1968).

The task of training adolescents for responsibility is a complex one. Help needs to be given in defining the problem, providing the necessary information (or where it can be found), and assisting in the process of weighing up and predicting the likely consequences of alternative choices. Next, the decision must really be the young person's who consequently must also be allowed to cope with its outcome. Then the adult should not interfere even if he disagrees with the choice made (unless the wrong decision would really be quite disastrous); at the same time he should be prepared to stand by the adolescent if things do go wrong and give what help he can in putting things right.

Just as at present too many children grow up without insight into their own feeling and motives, so many get the opportunity too rarely to make their own decisions with a clear awareness beforehand of what is involved and with the responsibility afterwards to accept the consequences. Yet only such understanding and such practice will eventually enable them to deal competently with their own emotions and with their own decisions.

Schools have a vital contribution to make here. In the conventional classroom setting, where both work and discipline are laid down by the teacher, there is relatively little room for allowing each child a measure of responsibility for his own actions and learning. A more pupil-centred regime gives children a sense of involvement and participation in planning their own activities according to their different interest and ability levels; while rules evolved jointly with the teacher help to make the reasons for necessary constraints understood and hence more readily accepted by the pupils.

Research has shown that schools which emphasise cooperation rather than competition, which neither stream nor use corporal punishment, have a lower incidence of bullying, violence and delinquency, without any lowering of academic standards. Also, fostering emotional and social potential may prove more conducive to improving a child's rate of learning than concentrating more directly but narrowly on educational progress itself (Gooch and Pringle, 1966; Marjoribanks, 1978; Rutter et al. 1979).

Many non-academic adolescents have for long felt that schooling is not sufficiently about life as they know it. This feeling has increasingly come to be shared by their grammar school peers and was well expressed by the sixth-former who edited *Youth Now* (Hadingham, 1970) when he wrote: 'Education is not simply a matter of passing exams and reaching university, but of playing a responsible, active part in social and political life.' This desire for a closer contact with 'real life' is a vital ingredient in the process of growing towards moral and emotional maturity. Young people are involved in a number of different and often interacting social groups – family, peer groups, school and society. Secondary schools could be playing a major role in helping adolescents to interpret themselves in relation to these groups and these groups in relation to themselves. To achieve this, a more appropriate curriculum must be devised.

Such a curriculum synthesises cognitive, emotional and moral aspects. Its appropriate setting is a school community in which the same principles of relationship and responsibility obtain as those included in the curriculum. To combine an appropriate curriculum with an appropriate school community opens up for the adolescent a rich developmental experience with which he can identify because he recognises what it offers as the means to his personal fulfilment (Hemming, 1974).

A BILL OF RIGHTS FOR CHILDREN?

Children's special needs have not been a major concern of our country. Child labor laws and universal education are related to industrialisation and a way to keep unneeded child workers out of the labor market but off the streets... What is necessary for the nurturance, even survival, of our democracy are child development programmes which use our present knowledge to facilitate the development of effective, responsible adults... The time is now for a stand on behalf of our children (Berlin, 1975).

The author then proposes a Bill of Rights for children which includes all the basic needs of children discussed in this chapter. Similarly it covers all the 'Rights of the Child' set out in the Children's Charter to which President Hoover's 1930 White House Conference pledged itself, but which still has not been accorded any priority for early implementation.

Is the situation in this country not very similar? Children have few rights in law; nor has the protection of their interests much more legal backing than in the United States; their voice is rarely heard and even more rarely taken into account in decisions affecting their well-being. Children's needs differ from adults', if only because the possibilities of improvement or of long-term damage are so much greater. Would not a Bill of Rights be a means of safeguarding their interests, at least to some extent?

3. The Parental and Family Role

The multi-generation family, which included a large number of children as well as grandparents – and possibly some other relatives – is held by many sociological, anthropological and historical writers to have been the pre-industrial, near-universal model. However, a recent study argues that the large extended family has in fact never been the norm, either in this country or in Western society (Laslett, 1972). It suggests that the large family is part of a kind of 'Golden Age ideology', which nostalgically prefers a mythical past to what society and life were actually like. From the late Middle Ages onwards, 'The nuclear family household constituted the ordinary, expected, normal framework of domestic existence ... It is simply untrue, as far as we can tell ... that the complex family was a universal background to the ordinary lives of ordinary people.'

What has perhaps changed is that most people no longer live near relatives and friends most of their lives, so that they are not surrounded by a network of kinship and neighbourhood, all within walking distance. Increased mobility has made for greater isolation, almost anonymity, in high density conditions of modern urban life. In what follows the parental role in the modern nuclear family will be considered within the context of Western societies.

Basically this consists of meeting the developmental needs of childhood – which vary, of course, with age – to ensure optimal growth of all a child's potentialities. Comparative studies of child-rearing methods have shown that the quality, type and amount of contact with parents and with other children all have a differential effect on development.

To begin with, it is primarily the inter-action between mother and infant which satisfies the basic physical and psychological needs. Evidence suggests that, to be maximally effective, it has to be a two-way process: not only does the child imitate the mother but the mother also imitates the child (Bell, 1968; Bronfenbrenner, 1970).

Thus, it is the one-to-one relationship and its continuing and reciprocal nature which promote maximal learning and progress.

Preparing the child for life outside the family home is one of the major social functions of the parental role. The quality of family relationships exerts a profound and lasting influence on children's psychological development. The family which is able and equipped to carry out its parental tasks consistently and successfully gives a sense of security, of companionship and belonging to each of its members; it also bestows a sense of purpose and direction, of achievement and of personal worth. For the child it is of unique importance because it mediates between him and the world at large, providing what might be called a buffer, a filter and a bridge. It thus fulfils the irreplaceable function of laying the basis for the adjustment of the individual within society. The capacity for integration, cooperation and creativity has its roots in family living.

PARENTING – A SHARED TASK

Lip service has for long been paid to the concept of parenting being a shared task. But even today, when many more fathers are involved with the birth and nurturing of their children, it remains common for men to exclude themselves from the birth and early months of their baby's life. Indeed, even psychological preparation for motherhood is still uncommon though relaxation classes – which may include talking about or demonstrating various tasks of mothering, such as bathing a baby or how to sterilise its bottle – have become increasingly widespread. Yet these months of waiting may well be an emotionally most receptive time for both partners. Surely the shared task of parenting could and should begin right at the beginning?

> Pregnancy and birth involve developmental crises, not only for the woman but very often for the man too (as well as for the larger family of which they are a part). It is a key point in their individual life cycle and in the cycle of their relationship, whether or not the couple are married. Education for childbirth and parenthood can help the prospective parents towards maturation . . . it can help towards a deeper understanding of relationships – between the couple and in-laws, between the parents and child – in the family and in the wider society (Kitzinger, 1973).

The next phase of parenting when sharing becomes particularly important is the post-natal period. A great deal of attention, joy and interest are focused on the mother and her new baby, but these tend to wane just when she is likely to be in greatest need of support, namely two or three months after the actual birth. By that time, the father is beginning to realise more fully the extent of his wife's preoccupation with the baby and its effect on their relationship. The young mother may be growing exhausted from her new responsibilities and anxieties, broken nights and perhaps feeding difficulties, made worse by feelings of social isolation and post-natal depression. These may engender anger, or even hatred and rejection, of the baby which in turn lead her to fear that she might do it some harm. It then becomes vital that she has support, understanding and counselling available to her, not only from her partner, relatives and friends but also from professional helpers (Pringle, 1980).

THE PATERNAL ROLE

The father's part in fostering the child's development is primarily a two-fold one: firstly, it provides the child with a second adult model so that he can identify with a member of his own sex, if a boy, and also learn at first hand about the behaviour and attitudes of the opposite sex, if a girl. Secondly, better developmental progress appears to be made when praise and recognition come not only from the mother but from another person, preferably of the opposite sex (Bronfenbrenner, 1970).

There is a third likelihood for which there is not yet research evidence: the mother herself probably receives reassurance in her maternal role from her husband's support so that he 'reinforces' not only the child's but her own feelings of adequacy and self-esteem; this in turn increases her confidence in her mothering which communicates itself to the child. The same may well be true in relation to the mother, conveying both to father and child the value of the paternal role (Pedersen, 1976).

There is also some evidence that children's sense of responsibility develops best not in a matriarchal or patriarchal family structure, but where both parents participate actively in child rearing with somewhat different roles: the father increasingly becoming the principal companion and disciplinarian for the boy as he grows older and the mother for the girl. The father's absence – particularly where it is for long periods or permanent – has been shown to have an unfavourable effect on the child's psychological development, especially when it happens during the pre-school years; the influence of the father's absence on the mother will also affect the child, both directly and indirectly (Pilling and Pringle, 1978).

Being a readily replaceable cog in the industrial machine deprives many a man of a sense of identity and personal value. To a considerable extent this loss could be restored to the breadwinner by the family. Fathers can make an indispensable contribution to the psychological development of their children, daughters as well as sons (Smith, 1980; Chibucos and Kail, 1981; Lamb, 1981). The importance of the mother–child relationship has been so much stressed in recent years that it almost seemed fathers need merely to provide material things for their offspring.

Work with handicapped children has shown how mistaken this view is. Where the father shares responsibility for upbringing and care, there is a much better chance of the child's triumphing over his disabilities than if the mother is left to cope by herself. The same is now seen to apply also to the normal child. 'For optimal development bonds need to be formed with people of both sexes and it is very likely that early attachments will influence the kind of close relationships which are possible later' (Rutter, 1981).

Through a true partnership with their wives, fathers can give a living example of democratic cooperation which their sons may then emulate and their daughters may seek in their future husbands. By taking an active part in his children's everyday care, finding time to play and later to share interests with them, fathers can enjoy and get to know them from their earliest age. Delegating it all to the mother until the children are older prevents the building up of those early relationships which are of such vital importance.

> In short, a three-person model, including two adults of the opposite sex, appears to be more effective for socialisation than a two-person mother-child model... The fact that the structure most conducive to a child's development turns out to be the family is hardly surprising. The family is, after all, the product of a million years of evolution and should therefore have some survival value for the species (Bronfenbrenner, 1973).

SHARING THE PARENTAL ROLE

Can parental care be given in settings different from conventional family life as we know it? Communes have not been established long enough to assess their effects on child development. The Israeli

Kibbutz is the only Western child-rearing pattern which is markedly different. Upbringing is shared from the earliest months of life between parents and professional educators, the latter undertaking the major part of the daily care, training, teaching and disciplining (Avgar et al., 1977).

Parental concern and involvement remain nevertheless paramount; the choice of the caring personnel, as well as the pattern of care, are decided by, and remain under the close surveillance of, the parents themselves; also each child spends three or more hours daily with his parents. During this time, they are free from all other responsibilities to devote their whole attention to playing with, talking to and enjoying their children. This is very different from the kind of half-attention given for part of or throughout the day in our society to pre-school children by mothers, busy with cleaning, shopping and cooking; and very different, too, from maternal or paternal separation.

Though it is nonsense to equate Kibbutz methods of child upbringing with maternal deprivation, this claim has nevertheless been made from time to time. In fact, it is a very specific way of dividing the parental role which is unique in developed societies. It is worth noting that over the years increasing responsibility has been given to mothers in most Kibbutzim for the care of their infants. For example, they now have six weeks off from work to nurse their newborn babies; and then they work half-time or less for a further six months, devoting the rest of the day entirely to the baby, since all work is done communally.

The evidence regarding the effects of a Kibbutz upbringing remains contradictory. There is said to be virtually no juvenile crime, few serious sexual difficulties, no homosexuality and practically no illegitimacy; also a disproportionately large number achieve high political office and high rank in the armed forces. So far, the Kibbutz has produced few major artists, writers or musicians; and, by American standards, young people are said to be over-dependent on the approval of their peers.

It is worthy of note that among the first generation of children, now themselves becoming parents, many wish their children to live in their own homes. Greater affluence makes this possible by simply enlarging the living space of each family. Youngsters themselves also want to sleep most nights with their own families, at least up to the age of twelve to fourteen years; then they begin to opt increasingly for sharing sleeping quarters with their contemporaries in the children's house.

SHARING MATERNAL ATTENTION

The only, as well as the first-born, child has an exceptional position in the family. On the one hand, he is more likely to be over-protected because his parents are relatively inexperienced; over-anxiety about development and progress may also be more common for the same reason. It is possible, too, that first-borns tend to be more competitive because they internalise their parents' high hopes for them; and jealousy of subsequent arrivals may also express itself in a desire to excel and beat competitors (including younger brothers and sisters).

On the other hand, the first-born does not have to compete for attention with siblings, at least to begin with; he is conceived and reared at a time when parental vigour, both physical and intellectual, is likely to be at its height; and the parents, but particularly the mother, have more time and energy to devote to him throughout the time during which he remains an only child. Any of these factors may be expected to promote the fullest realisation of a first child's potentiality, not least because he is given a headstart during his early life (White et al., 1979).

There is agreement in the literature that 'the dice are loaded in favour of the first-born' (Hudson, 1970). That this is so has been demonstrated again by a recent study of infants during their first year of life, and also by the Bureau's *National Child Development Study*. The former compared the effects of being reared in three different environments in Israel, namely family, Kibbutz and residential institution. Attention was concentrated on only children and the youngest child in a family. The same type of behaviour, namely vocalisation and smiling, was observed in both the infants and in those looking after them.

As one would have predicted, the adults spoke and smiled least in the institutional setting, and most often in the family; only children were spoken to and smiled at markedly more often than the youngest in the family; in the Kibbutz, the frequency was comparable to that of mothers in the family in relation to the youngest child. All these differences were mirrored in the infants themselves (Gewirtz and Gewirtz, 1969).

Since results from the Bureau's *National Child Development Study* will be quoted from time to time by way of illustration, a brief description of its design and aims might be useful. It is based on the Perinatal Mortality Survey, the subjects of which consisted of a whole week's births, some 17,000 babies in all, born in the week 3–9 March 1958, in England, Scotland and Wales. An unparalleled amount of sociological, obstetric and medical information was collected concerning the mother and the course of her pregnancy and labour, as well as detailed information on the baby at the time of delivery; a record was also made of the infant's weight, progress and any illnesses in the first weeks of life (Butler and Bonham, 1963; Butler and Alberman, 1969).

In 1965 (and also in 1969, 1974 and 1981) it proved possible to trace and study again the children and young people who as babies had been the survivors of the Perinatal Mortality Survey. This longitudinal follow-up investigation is called the *National Child Development Study*. At each follow-up, detailed information has been gathered from four main sources. First, a comprehensive picture was obtained from the schools of each pupil's abilities, behaviour and adjustment as well as about the school itself and about the contact between school and home.

Secondly, mothers, and sometimes fathers too, provided information about the home environment as well as about the child's development and behaviour. Thirdly, from a special medical examination, data were gathered on the children's height, weight, speech, hearing, vision, coordination and laterality. And fourthly, each child was given a number of tests and assessments (Pringle, Butler and Davie, 1966; Davie, Butler and Goldstein, 1972; Donnison, 1972).

Children with special needs too, such as those who are born illegitimate, adopted, handicapped, socially disadvantaged or gifted, have been studied (Crellin, Pringle and West, 1971; Seglow, Pringle and Wedge, 1972; Hitchfield, 1973; Wedge and Prosser, 1973; Ferri, 1976; Essen, 1979; Lambert and Streather, 1980; Essen and Wedge, 1982; Walker, 1982; Fogelman, 1983; Ferri, 1984; Shepherd, 1985).

The *NCDS* explored the question of shared maternal attention in two ways: firstly, in relation to family size, and secondly in relation to working mothers whose children are cared for during part of the day. The results of the former investigation show that even at birth family size begins to exert an influence, high perinatal mortality being associated with high parity. By 7–11, the overall picture clearly indicates that children from large families are at a considerable disadvantage physically, educationally and in terms of social adjustment.

For example, not only are children with many siblings shorter than those with few, but the arrival of each additional child also appears to act subsequently as a check to the growth of all preceding, i.e., older children; so, when there are younger siblings, the first-born does not reach the height of an only child at the age of seven or eleven years. In reading, the difference in attainment between the first and the fourth, or later born children was equivalent to sixteen months of reading age, and two or more younger children had an additional 'effect' of seven months. Conversely, those in one- or two-child families were about twelve months advanced in reading compared with those in families of five or more children (Davie, Butler and Goldstein, 1972; Prosser, 1973). These findings are very much in line with those of other studies of the effects of family size (Wadsworth, 1979).

It is not solely a question of low income, and thus a lower standard of living, since these effects of family size upon development were found to operate irrespective of social class. Obviously one explanation is that when parental time, attention, and maybe also patience, have to be shared, less is available for each child; this appears to be as true in respect of psychological resources as it is in terms of the family budget.

The child of the working mother shares the mother's attention with whatever paid responsibility she undertakes. To the extent that she has less time available to interact with and stimulate him, one might have expected a similar 'effect' to that of family size. However, this was not found to be so to the same extent (Davie, Butler and Goldstein, 1972; Wedge, 1973; Pilling and Pringle, 1978).

For example, after allowing for social class and family size, the average reading level of those whose mothers started work before the commencement of compulsory schooling was only three months below those whose mothers did not work; and where mothers started work after the child went to school, the difference shrank to six weeks. The effects were rather less if the work was on a part-time basis. In any case, it is likely that it is not so much the mother's working outside the home which affects the child's development as the quality of the substitute care which she is able to arrange.

PARENTS' INVOLVEMENT WITH THEIR CHILDREN

Relatively limited evidence is available on this aspect of parenthood. Much remains to be learned about the influence of the home background and of family relationships on child development; and about exactly how parental behaviour and expectations interact with the growing personality. Considerably more is known about the consequences of inadequate than of satisfactory parenting, most likely because 'happy families have no history' (Tolstoy, *Anna Karenina*).

While there is general agreement that the child's relationship with his parents is of vital importance, there have been a few voices of dissent regarding the most propitious nature of this relationship. For example, Musgrove (1966) argues that if it is

> close, warm and affectionate, the child is likely to be handicapped for life...The boy's long-term interests are best served by an inadequate and feckless (if 'demanding') father...to be left alone is perhaps one of the most urgent needs of children in a child- and home-centred society.

In fact, among the upper middle classes in Britain in the nineteenth and early part of the twentieth century, parental involvement with children was quite circumscribed, being delegated first to nannies and then to boarding schools. That this markedly affected emotional and social development is strongly suggested by available evidence which, however, is mainly biographical and autobiographical. There is even less evidence on the effects of the nanny's modern substitute, the *au pair* girl; it may well have even greater disadvantages, since she lacks both training and permanency. Furthermore, many know very little English, at least to begin with. Most are themselves young and may have little understanding of a small child's needs. Perhaps worst of all, since they usually stay for a few months only, the child suffers the bewildering, if not traumatic, experience of being looked after by a succession of such girls who inevitably bring with them the differing expectations and habits of their own national cultures.

Musgrove's views, however, have received little supportive evidence and are diametrically opposed to conclusions based on examining child-rearing practices in the United States as well as those based on cross-cultural studies (Bronfenbrenner, 1970; Devereux, Bronfenbrenner and Rodgers, 1969). There has been, it is argued, 'a decrease in all spheres of inter-action between parents and children . . . Over recent decades, children have been receiving progressively less attention . . . As parents and other adults have moved out of the lives of children, the vacuum has been filled by the age-segregated peer group.' It might also be that the radio and, even more, television have played a part in filling this vacuum, both here and in other developed countries.

Bronfenbrenner contends that in this trend of decreasing inter-action are to be found the roots of the growing alienation of children and youth in American society; and that, as a matter of urgency, policies and programmes should be planned to upgrade the role and functions of parenthood, to foster community involvement, to re-integrate children and schools into the life of the neighbourhood and to give genuine responsibility to youth for the care of the young. These proposals are very much in line with suggestions which have also been put forward in this country in recent years (Halsey, 1973; Leissner et al., 1971; Pringle, 1980; Ward, 1978).

THE PARAMOUNTCY OF 'BIOLOGICAL' PARENTHOOD AND THE MYTH OF MATERNAL FULFILMENT

On this question of paramountcy, society's attitude in this country is ambivalent and contradictory. Both in law and in practice we often act as if the blood tie and natural parenthood ensure satisfactory parenting. Yet, on the one hand, we fail to provide sufficient community support to enable parents to look after their children in times of difficulty; for example, every year several thousand pre-school children suffer the distress of coming into local authority care because their mothers are giving birth to another baby.

On the other hand, we so over-value the child's ties with his natural family that we let him remain with patently disturbed or rejecting parents. For example, a baby who has been assaulted and injured is allowed to return to his home in the hope that social work support will avoid a recurrence, when both common sense and research indicate that there is a high chance of it happening again. All the more so since social services are rarely, if ever, in a position to provide the daily surveillance required if a recurrence is to be prevented.

To argue that the parent needs the baby for his or her own recovery is to sacrifice the child's welfare to that of the adult. It was estimated in 1970 that around 700 infants were dying each year in England and Wales as a result of physical assault, and though since then the number has decreased it is still appallingly high. The number of children suffering non-fatal physical assault in 1982, sometimes involving permanent brain damage or crippling, has been estimated at over 6,000 (Creighton, 1984). 'The depth of suffering is extreme and, tragically, is perpetuated from generation to generation. Battered children grow up to batter their own babies' (Jobling, 1975). Those who come to official notice may be only the tip of the iceberg. Moreover, excessive stress is not invariably the cause as tends to be claimed. (Smith et al., 1973; Oliver and Cox, 1973; Smith et al., 1974; Franklin, 1977; Pringle, 1981, D.H.S.S., 1982; Lynch and Roberts, 1982).

There is also a contemporary myth about the effects which fulfilling the maternal role has upon a single girl who has herself been rejected in childhood. It is argued that she should not be offered birth control facilities or later advised to have her baby adopted despite her own immaturity and emotional inadequacy. Rather, it is said that when her need to have something which belongs to her is fullfilled by having a baby, she will grow to greater maturity and stability.

In fact there is no evidence whatever to support this assumption of a therapeutic effect. On the contrary, available clinical and casework material shows that there is a high probability of the baby's coming into care within the first year or two of its life; even if he returns to his mother from time to time, or remains with her, his chances in life are unfavourable practically from conception onwards (see Chapter 6, p. 125).

Again, the child's welfare is being sacrificed to that of the adult. It is a disturbing reflection of current attitudes to parenthood that one study has found one third of pregnancies among women who enjoy a stable relation with a man to have been unwanted; and that half of these unwanted pregnancies remained regretted (Office of Population Censuses and Surveys, 1973).

If the quality of children's lives is to be improved, then several notions need to be dispelled which have no foundation in fact: that having a child is the sole or most important or easiest way to feminine fulfilment (many a dissatisfied woman is doomed to disappointment and, worse still, may then come to resent the baby for failing to bring this fulfilment); that a baby completes a family, rather like a T.V. set or fridge; that it will cement a failing marriage; and that a child belongs to his parents like their other possessions over which they may exercise exclusive rights. At most, he is theirs only on temporary loan, as it were. There needs to be a shift from stressing the importance of parental rights to an emphasis on parental duties; and from the child being regarded as a chattel to a recognition of his right to loving care. The current idealised picture of parenthood needs to be replaced by a realistic and perhaps even daunting image of the arduous demands it imposes on one's emotions, energy, time and finance, as well as the inevitable constraints on personal independence, freedom of movement and indeed one's whole way of life.

It is evident that the ability and willingness to undertake all these responsibilities is neither dependent, nor necessarily consequent, upon biological parenthood. Rather it is the single-minded, unconditional desire, together with the emotional maturity to provide a caring home, which is the hallmark of good parenting.

MOTHERHOOD BY CHOICE

How are women – and men for that matter too – to tell whether they are really cut out for parenthood; whether they possess the unselfishness, patience, sensitivity and physical stamina to cope with all its demands? Preparation for parenthood – a practical appreciation of what is involved – should be an essential part of the curriculum for all children, more vital than sex or political education (Pringle, 1980).

In addition, women should no longer be subjected to the twin social pressures to marry and have children, yet to feel they are 'wasting their education' or are otherwise 'unfulfilled' if they devote themselves full-time to child-care. While it was the destiny of yesterday's woman to raise a family, today it can be her choice. Henceforth only those willing to devote some years to this task should contemplate it; and they should then receive recognition for undertaking one of the most crucial tasks for society's future. Motherhood by choice is in itself likely to improve its status. The fact that for the first time in sixty years there are now more males than females in the U.K. will also make for quite profound changes in the attitudes of each sex towards the other as well as towards parenthood.

4. Behaviour Problems and Learning Difficulties

Growing up is a difficult, and at times rather unhappy, business because of the child's very lack of experience: the younger he is, the more exclusively he lives in the present and the less he can draw comfort from a sense of perspective as well as from the knowledge, which time alone can bring, that most anxieties and problems are transitory.

However much parents try to protect their child from frightening situations, however reasonable and loving they may be, however child-centred a school they choose for him, growing up is inevitably beset by difficulties. Learning to manage feelings, learning to make sense of a bewilderingly complex world and learning to find one's own identity, bring both joy and sadness. Hence, all children find it difficult from time to time to adjust to the demands and expectations of the adult world. What then is the difference between children with problems and problem children?

THE CONCEPT OF MALADJUSTMENT

Hard and fast distinctions between 'normal' and 'abnormal' behaviour are artificial since the difference is one of degree and not of kind: the maladjusted child closely resembles the normal child in the way he reacts to insecurity, jealousy, rejection, inconsistent handling, or whatever it may be; but he shows these reactions in an intensified form.

All children pass through phases of temporary maladjustment. Transient problem behaviour is so common as to be normal and it has in fact been argued that a child who has never shown any difficulties should be considered abnormal. The negativistic three-year-old who has made 'no' and 'shan't' his most frequently used phrases; the seven-year-old who is anxious about going into the big junior school; the thirteen-year-old who is moody and inconsistent –

these reactions are characteristic of a particular age and stage of development.

CRITERIA POINTING TO MALADJUSTMENT

Five criteria might be found helpful when considering problem behaviour. The first criterion is chronological age, which means viewing a child's behaviour in the light of developmental norms. Frequent temper tantrums are quite common in a four-year-old, are unusual in a seven-year-old, but are so rare in an eleven-year-old that at that age they are likely to indicate serious disturbance.

The second criterion is intelligence. Age alone is insufficient for judging the significance of behaviour which deviates from what is usual for a particular age group. For example, the eight-year-old who prefers his own company or that of adults to his contemporaries; who refuses to learn by rote; who will not admit defeat and cries angrily when unable to solve a problem he has set himself; who refuses to go to sleep because he never has enough time to complete what he wants to do; who is insatiably curious and bitterly resents interruptions; such a child is clearly out of step with those of his own age. However, when it becomes recognised that his intelligence (or, as some people prefer to call it, his educable capacity) is similar to that of the average twelve-year-old, then his behaviour is seen to be part of a general developmental acceleration rather than symptomatic of emotional disturbance. Of course, high intellectual ability and maladjustment are not mutually exclusive.

The third and fourth criteria are the intensity and the persistence of a particular symptom. For example, a good many children have fears, tell lies and steal. Emotional difficulties must be suspected when a child is so full of fears that no sooner does one disappear than another takes its place; or when he persists in fabricating, and believing in, fantastic stories long after most children have learned to distinguish between fact and fiction.

An example showing the significance of the intensity of a symptom might be nailbiting. Research has shown that the great majority of children bite their nails at some time or other. However, few do it to the extent of drawing blood. Such a degree of intensity indicates emotional disturbance rather than just a bad habit; another example is the child who seems quite unable to tell the truth, even when it would be to his advantage.

The fifth criterion is a child's home background, including its cultural and social setting. For example, Jean lived in a high-delinquency area; her family had a criminal record, unusually consistent even in such a district (both parents, three brothers and one sister having been in prison, borstal and approved schools respectively); by coming into conflict with the law, Jean followed the family pattern. Her delinquencies were unlikely to be symptoms of maladjustment but rather reflected a lack of moral and social training. This in no way implies that such antisocial behaviour should be condoned; rather that the measures needed for re-education and rehabilitation will be different from those appropriate for the maladjusted child. In contrast, when twelve-year-old John, the son of a headmaster, spent his leisure time breaking open gas meters, this activity was the outward expression of strong inner conflicts, since such behaviour was out of keeping with his family's standards and the social and moral training given to him.

On the one hand, just as nature allows wide individual variations in physical stamina, so it probably does with respect to emotional stability. For example, individual differences in such traits as fear and affection are quite evident in the first year or two of life. Even the Dionne quins, who were biologically similar and brought up almost identically, showed individual differences in social development by the time they were two years old.

On the other hand, there is ample evidence – from clinical, sociological and psychological work – that a great deal of emotional maladjustment is related to, if not caused by, an unfavourable home or school environment. Lack of sufficient insight and support on the part of parents or teachers may be decisive factors in whether or not a child is able to cope with stressful situations. The belief that 'there are no problem children, only problem parents or teachers' is supported by the fact that emotional difficulties may clear up completely after help has been given.

Since there is constant interaction from conception onwards between hereditary and environmental influences, it is quite impossible in any given case to attribute difficulties solely to one or the other, or to apportion the extent to which either factor is responsible. For example, a boy may have inherited his father's quick temper and irritability; excessive aggressiveness may, however, equally well be due to being continually subjected to outbursts of temper, coupled with the fact that boys tend to identify themselves with their fathers. In practice, emphasising the influence of heredity may well become a self-fulfilling prophecy.

A more constructive attitude lies in placing the main emphasis on the positive influence which environment can exert at any stage of a child's development. This means acting on the assumption that problem behaviour is due to adverse factors in the family or social environment or in the child's own make-up; but that, given help, at least some readjustment can take place by redirecting such behaviour into more constructive channels.

CONFLICT AND LEARNING

'Children must be allowed to do as they please, as conflict causes problem behaviour.' This fallacy is unfairly attributed to the teaching of modern psychology. Conflict is essential to growth. It only becomes harmful when it poses a problem which is insoluble or which is inappropriate to the child's age and ability.

Indeed, for any development to take place, the child must learn to give up more primitive behaviour for new, more mature satisfactions. For example, the two-year-old has to give up the comfort of being carried about, for the pleasure of independent locomotion; the five-year-old must inhibit the inclination to grab what he wants, for the advantage of playing cooperatively with others; the thirteen-year-old must resolve the conflict between joining the leisure activities of his friends and doing homework, which will earn him the approval of parents and teachers or better marks or whatever satisfaction is most desired at the time. Of course, a conflict will not invariably be solved in the more mature direction but then progress rarely proceeds in a straight line.

The harm comes from inappropriate or insoluble conflict, the more so if it is chronic. A two-year-old cannot be expected to give up grabbing for the sake of sharing with others nor can the five-year-old be expected to choose doing homework instead of playing; and there is no satisfactory solution open to the child who is unwanted or whose loyalties are being competed for by warring parents who openly disagree about his upbringing. Such conflicts undermine a child's sense of security and impede healthy growth because no constructive alternatives are available.

THE MEANING AND SIGNIFICANCE OF SYMPTOMS

Just like pain, symptoms of maladjustment are a danger signal, a call for help; they indicate that there is intolerable tension between the personality and the environment. Withdrawal is as urgent a danger signal as aggression although the latter is more likely to be heeded because it constitutes a threat to adult authority. The range of possible symptoms is wide but basically they fall into two broad categories: aggression or withdrawal, fight or flight. Some children habitually choose one mode of reaction, others oscillate between retreat and attack.

To some extent, habitual behaviour is determined by personality type. The emotionally robust, confident and outgoing child is likely to adopt outgoing, aggressive methods whilst the gentle and retiring one is likely to choose retreat. To begin with, a child will try out various means of meeting a difficult situation. Experience then teaches him which is the most effective or least painful way.

Thus the relative success of aggressive or withdrawn behaviour influences which facet of the child's personality subsequently finds predominant expression. If he gains his ends more readily by one mode, he will persevere with this behaviour pattern. Hence, the way in which the earliest attempts at non-conformity and independence are handled has a vital influence on shaping later reactions to adult authority. By the time a child begins school the decisive choice between aggression and withdrawal has usually been made and the same choice is likely to be made in the school situation. This is one more reason why purely educational or purely emotional problems are rarely found in practice.

In practice, nuisance value or social unacceptability still tend to be used as the main criteria of problem behaviour. This leads to two undesirable consequences: the aggressive child who hits back arouses aggression in the adults concerned; this leads to a vicious circle of increasingly severe punishment calling out increasing aggression in the child who grows hardened to punishment, so that it loses its effectiveness. Secondly, the withdrawn, over-conforming child, though receiving gentler handling, tends to be overlooked. His real needs are likely to remain unmet since the understanding that a child can be 'too good' is still slow in coming.

No generally acceptable definition exists of a mentally healthy child; however, there would probably be general agreement that a confident, enquiring attitude of mind and the ability to make mutually rewarding relationships, both with adults and peers, are essential characteristics. Viewed in this context, the anxious, timid, always obedient child must cause concern. In fact, fight or flight, aggression or withdrawal, need to be regarded as equally significant danger signs, indicating that a child's emotional, social or intellectual needs are not being adequately met.

Symptoms of maladjustment are perhaps most appropriately likened to a fever: a sign of malaise, of disease, indicating the need for careful examination and diagnosis but by itself providing little clue to what is wrong or to effective treatment. Knowing the symptoms does not provide the key to the underlying causes; nor does knowing the underlying causes make it possible to predict likely symptoms.

Take, for example, stealing: parental rejection was the underlying cause with Ann; her parents wanted a boy and instead had a girl, and a rather timid and plain one at that. Peter, on the other hand, subjected to harsh discipline by his ex-sergeant-major father, expressed his defiance by stealing; and in Edward's case, stealing was not so much a symptom of maladjustment as due to a feckless home where he lacked moral guidance. Thus the same symptom may have a variety of causes. Hence action appropriate in one case would be inapplicable, ineffective, and possibly even harmful, in another.

Conversely, the same underlying causes may find expression in different symptoms. For example, Alan, jealous of his brilliant, popular brother, reacted by over-conformity, timidity, bed-wetting and underfunctioning at school; while Jennifer, faced with the same problem of jealousy, was spiteful and disobedient at home, but at school was over-ambitious and extremely hardworking. Thus the actual symptoms shown were almost diametrically opposed.

THE CONCEPT OF UNDERACHIEVEMENT

The term 'backwardness' relates educational attainment to chronological age, and hence to the level of work reached by the majority of a child's contemporaries; underachievement or underfunctioning relate it to the capacity of the individual pupil. In the one case a group norm serves as the yardstick, in the other it is the learning ability of the particular child in question.

The needs of children who are either educationally backward, slow learning or both, have received considerable attention in recent years. Though provision to meet their needs still remains inadequate, at least they are fairly well understood. This is by no means the case with regard to underachievement. Far too often it is still thought – by parents and even by teachers – that if a child does badly at school he must be either stupid, lazy or possibly both; large classes and inexperienced teachers are also made to take a share of the blame.

That intellectually able or very able children may in their schoolwork not reach the level of their own potential, or fail to achieve even the level of the majority of their own age group, is an idea which has been particularly slow in gaining acceptance despite available evidence (Pringle, 1970).

Exceptionally intelligent children can hardly be expected to function at a level commensurate with their mental age. For one thing, it is unlikely that they will be taught at so advanced a stage; for another, it is by no means established that the teaching appropriate for the average fifteen-year-old is equally suitable – qualitatively or quantitatively – for the ten-year-old who has a mental age of fifteen years. Moreover, for the most outstandingly gifted, such as a mathematical genius, the commonly used standards of attainment are anyhow unlikely to be applicable. Be that as it may, the education of able children generally, and the needs of able underfunctioning children in particular, have so far received only limited consideration in Britain.

CAUSES OF EDUCATIONAL DIFFICULTIES

Because of the close link between emotion and learning, scholastic failure is often accompanied by behaviour difficulties of one kind or another. Since the basis of all learning is laid in the home during the earliest years of life, the chances are high that, in many cases, the roots of educational difficulties may also be found there.

These conclusions have been confirmed once again by the findings from the *National Child Development Study*. For example, the incidence of maladjustment at the age of seven was four times higher among poor readers than among the rest of the cohort. By seven, children have been at school long enough for backwardness in reading to be reliably assessed but not so long that their difficulties are likely to have led to maladjustment in any but a few cases, particularly since most infant schools do not 'label' or otherwise penalise the slower learner. This strongly suggests that maladjustment is often a cause or at least an accompaniment of backwardness rather than a result of it (Davie et al., 1972).

The parents' attitudes to the child, to achievement in general and to scholastic success in particular, as well as their own level of education and the cultural stimulation they provided during the pre-school years and thereafter, play a major part. The child's own personality and how he interacts with all environmental influences will determine his readiness, adaptation and responsiveness to the school situation.

This in turn may be favourable or inimical to his particular needs. If he is fortunate it will build on and supplement what his home has given him so far, thus extending his range of emotional relationships as well as his intellectual horizons. At worst, it may extinguish his curiosity and his delight in learning, because of an uninspired teaching approach, because there is failure in personal relations, or because of a combination of these.

The teacher who sees his role in a wider framework than the inculcating of skills and the purveying of information is in a position of great influence. He can counteract, or at least mitigate, some of the consequences of an emotionally or culturally unfavourable home background; he can rekindle the child's curiosity, harness his emotional energies by giving praise and recognition, and compensate him for emotional deprivation by offering affection, albeit of a less 'exclusive' and close nature than parental love. Of course, the larger the class and the more deprived the child, the more difficult it is for the teacher to give the necessary time and attention to an individual pupil. In most cases, it would also be essential to involve the parents and influence their attitudes.

The environmental factors leading to under-achievement or indeed 'over-achievement' will repay closer scrutiny and study. A genetically potential I.Q. of 150 is of little value to society if largely unused. Real equality of educational opportunity is a will-o'-the-wisp while inequality remains in the home. And by inequality in the home we do not especially imply an inequality in material factors but also, and perhaps more powerfully, an inequality in attitudes to the child, attitudes to education and attitudes to life which in combination appear to exert continuous and long term influences upon psychological growth. These inequalities do not merely reflect the differing practices of different social classes but also occur within classes, and indeed also appear to occur within families (Clarke and Clarke, 1972).

MULTIPLICITY OF CAUSATION

Perhaps most fundamental of all is the fact that rarely, if ever, are either problem behaviour or learning difficulties due to one single cause or circumstance. Rather there is a multiplicity of inter-related and inter-acting factors, so that there is unlikely to be a short cut either to diagnosis or to treatment. The health, appearance, intelligence and whole personality of the child; the economic, social and cultural standing of his parents; the relationship between them and between all the other members of the family; the child's experiences at school and in the neighbourhood – all these and many more factors may play a part. Their combination and impact are unique for each child. Thus the relative importance of a particular set of circumstances differs for each child, even in the same family, as does the aspect most likely to respond to intervention or therapy.

Frequently one is faced with the apparent paradox of one child who has survived an extremely unfavourable environment, apparently unscathed, while another has succumbed to far less adverse circumstances. The answer lies probably in the fact that the constitutionally most stable and resilient are capable of overcoming even intense and prolonged stress. Yet, everyone has a breaking point. The child's more malleable personality is more vulnerable and hence more likely to become irreparably warped than that of the mature adult. In addition to inborn differences in temperamental stability and intellectual potential, every child's development is helped or hindered by the opportunities afforded by his home and school to make appropriate choices and to cope with resolvable conflicts.

Perhaps an analogy might help to illustrate the way in which multiple causation accounts for learning and behaviour difficulties in childhood. Cars come in all shapes and sizes: some, like Land Rovers, can negotiate the roughest ground: others are so flimsily made that even relatively minor bumps in the road will soon lead to trouble; others yet are excellent of their kind, such as the Rolls-Royce, though not designed to travel over unmade country roads. Secondly, roads themselves not only differ, but become unexpectedly hazardous from time to time, due to floods, subsidence or other 'acts of God'.

Thirdly, drivers differ not only in their actual driving skills but also in their understanding, and indeed interest in, what makes the engine tick; some will do reasonably well given straightforward weather and road conditions; some will excel whatever the conditions; and others will be a hazard to themselves and other road users because of poor road sense, too slow or too fast reactions and a lack of understanding of what it is reasonable to expect from the particular model they are driving. Indeed, the majority of accidents are caused by human short-comings rather than by faults in the car's design, performance or capability.

For cars now substitute children: some are born sturdy and resilient; others are vulnerable, perhaps due to genetic factors or some slight neurological impairment but more often because of unsatisfactory life experiences which leave them inadequately equipped to cope with subsequent stress; a small minority are born actually damaged. For the road substitute life, which for the majority will be reasonably smooth with only occasional 'bumps' but for some may bring difficulties if not disaster.

Lastly, for the driver substitute parents and teachers. No one questions that the best made, reliable car can become a menace in the hands of an inexperienced, vacillating, selfish, impulsive, aggressive, neglectful, or simply stupid and generally inadequate driver. Nor that the highly skilled, responsible motorist takes his task seriously, devoting time and thought to obtaining the best performance his vehicle is capable of, and giving constant care to appropriate handling and servicing.

Of course, neither parents nor teachers deliberately mishandle children – the vast majority are deeply caring and concerned. But why is it assumed that because we have all been children, we know how best to foster the development of our own offspring? Most people would not accept the similar argument that because we have all been to school we could therefore be adequate teachers without the need for lengthy professional training. Though analogies must not be pushed too far, some preparation for parenthood seems desirable to bring about a much wider awareness and understanding of the developmental needs of children.

5. Consequences of Failure to Meet Children's Needs

If one of the basic needs remains unmet – or inadequately met – then development may become stunted or distorted. In practice it is likely that if one need fails to be met, others will be affected too, but in what follows the likely consequences will be discussed separately. It is also probable that there is an optimal level of need fulfilment so that 'too much' may also be harmful. This question will also be considered, but more briefly.

'We've tried everything'. . .'We treat them all alike'. . .'We've given the child everything he wants'. These three remarks are frequently heard when parents ask for help with a difficult child. The first suggests inconsistent handling, with swings between strict control and weak indulgence...The second overlooks the fact that siblings are not 'all alike' but vary in age and personality – and therefore in their individual needs...The third remark suggests that the parents have tried to compensate in irrelevant, extravagant material ways for their difficulty in meeting the child's emotional needs (Berry, 1972).

THE NEED FOR LOVE AND SECURITY

When this need is not met adequately, then the consequences can be disastrous later on, both for the individual and for society. Prisons, mental hospitals, borstals and schools for the maladjusted contain a high proportion of individuals who in childhood lacked consistent, continuous and concerned care, or, worse still, were unloved and rejected. Their number is high too among the chronically unemployable and among what I have termed 'able misfits' (Pringle, 1970).

Such young people are one example of the fact that parental rejection is neither the prerogative of any social class nor necessarily linked with socio-economic disadvantage. The existence of an unwanted child may more readily come to light in families whose other problems have already necessitated some involvement of one helping agency or another. In the affluent middle or upper class home, emotional deprivation is rarely suspected or detected; to the discerning teacher the signs are quite evident yet not infrequently it is the child himself who is blamed for his difficult behaviour and lack of progress, being labelled 'uncooperative', 'disruptive', 'lazy' or 'backward'.

Anger, hate and lack of concern for others are probable reactions to being unloved and rejected. Vandalism, violence and delinquency are not infrequently an outward expression of these feelings. In embryo these reactions can be seen when a young child, who has been scolded or smacked, kicks his teddy bear or the table. Through a loving relationship, children learn to control their anger and later to use it constructively during adolescence and adulthood; without affection, it remains primitive and grows more vicious and vengeful with increasing strength.

Can too much love and security be given to a child? There is a sense in which this may be so where a parent builds such a close and exclusive tie that eventual emancipation from it or even sharing it may not come about. As a result, the chance of future emotional independence may be jeopardised, together with the establishment of mutually satisfying sexual and parental relationships. Too much security – being as it were wrapped protectively in cotton wool – may make a child too fearful to venture out and face the uncertainties of a less safe and protective world.

Not so long ago it was believed that children became attached to their mothers chiefly because they provided nourishment. This theory of 'cupboard love' has been disproved by the work of the Harlows with monkeys and by Bowlby's studies of attachment behaviour. Now the pendulum may have swung so far in the other direction that there is a risk of the importance of nutrition being overlooked within this context. Recent evidence suggests that impaired food intake is probably an important contributory cause of dwarfism in children from neglectful or rejecting homes.

The concept of maternal deprivation

Bowlby's monograph, prepared for the World Health Organisation in 1951 on maternal deprivation, was a major landmark and his subsequent work has continued to shed light on the nature of mothering. The numerous studies carried out since then, both with humans and animals, bear witness to the remarkable influence of his thinking.

The contention, which Bowlby made his own, that the nature of the child's earliest emotional relationship to his mother is of vital importance; that he needs to establish a lasting 'bond'; and if it is irrevocably broken or has never been satisfactorily established, then subsequent physical, intellectual and social development may be seriously and lastingly affected, is now generally accepted; as is the evidence that if a child has not had the opportunity to become closely attached to one and the same mother-figure during the first three years of life, he may become a psychopath or 'affectionless character'.

Controversy has, however, continued to surround his views. Three aspects in particular have been challenged. First, that deprivation of maternal care inevitably causes permanent damage; for example, it is argued that mental retardation can be mitigated by appropriate training in later childhood despite severe deprivation in infancy (Clarke and Clarke, 1973). Secondly, it has been questioned whether all children are equally vulnerable to the distorting effects of such deprivation; indeed, Bowlby himself said that only some children are gravely damaged for life. There are likely to be innate differences in responsiveness to stress; equally important, there is evidence that the child's age and stage of development, as well as the degree and duration of maternal deprivation, are of crucial importance (Pringle, 1971).

Thirdly, it has been argued that the term itself is imprecise. It suggests that there has been a loss, when in many cases the child has never experienced continuous, loving care, i.e., he has always lacked it; in other cases the quality of care has been insufficient or distorted; if a relationship was established, it may have been interrupted for longer or shorter periods. Each of these situations is likely to have different effects on development; as is also the nature of the mother-child relationship prior to the separation experiences.

Incidentally, the question of love and security is invariably discussed within the context of the mother-child relationship because this is the usual situation in developed countries. However, there is no evidence that – if the mother went out to work – the father could not meet this need and bring up children equally well, given appropriate attitudes, both on his and on society's part. One would then expect prolonged paternal deprivation early in a child's life to have similar consequences to maternal deprivation.

In his reassessment of 'maternal deprivation', Rutter (1972) suggests that the concept

> should now be abandoned. That 'bad' care of children in early life can have 'bad' effects, both short-term and long-term, can be accepted as proven. What is now needed is a more precise delineation of the different aspects of 'badness', together with the analysis of their separate effects and the reasons why children differ in their responses.

Whether it is wise to give up this concept until there has been the further research that Rutter pleads for and until more discriminating terms become available, might be questioned.

In the writer's opinion it is more urgent to dispel two misconceptions which have had very unfortunate consequences. Both are based on misinterpretations of Bowlby's views. His stress on the need for a warm, intimate and continuous relationship has been taken to imply that the same person must provide care uninterruptedly for twenty-four hours a day. In fact, he has always held that it is wise to accustom even quite young babies to being looked after by someone else occasionally; yet some mothers continue to feel guilty about seeking a temporary and brief 'escape'.

The second misconception is seen in the dictum 'better a bad family than a good institution'. While there is no evidence to support this assertion, it has led to some official reluctance to remove children even from appallingly bad homes. This view ignores the most crucial factors in mothering, namely its quality, stability and intensity. Instead it postulates a powerful bond, commonly referred to as the 'blood tie'. Again, there is no evidence for this myth. Rather, present knowledge indicates that good mothering (or fathering for that matter) is neither dependent on, nor necessarily consequent upon, biological parenthood.

That this is so is shown by the generally very satisfactory outcome when children are placed in adoptive homes. Moreover, there is much evidence that this is the case even when a child has, prior to placement, been subjected to potentially damaging experiences, such as prenatal stress, early institutional care, parental neglect, ill-treatment, or even a combination of these (Kadushin, 1970; Pringle, 1966; Seglow, Pringle and Wedge, 1972; Skeels, 1966; Skodak and Skeels, 1949; Tizard, 1977).

The effects of maternal deprivation

Inevitably, the evidence for the relationship of maternal care to children's mental health comes primarily from two sources: from the clinical observations of those concerned with emotionally disturbed children; and from retrospective psychological studies which compare the development of family-reared children with those growing up deprived of a loving and secure home. Methodologically it would certainly be more conclusive if objective studies of intra-family behaviour in the 'natural' environment of the home were possible; clearly they are not. Controlled experiments to explore the effects of various types of maternal deprivation on human babies are, of course, quite unacceptable.

Just such experiments, however, have been carried out on baby monkeys. The results are clear cut, startling and convincing. Several generations of monkeys were raised under a wide range of depriving conditions: partial or complete deprivation of maternal care; rearing in complete isolation; rearing with other motherless infants; and varying the onset of these abnormal situations. This work was continued long enough to see whether infant experiences have effects lasting into adulthood (Harlow and Griffin, 1965; Harlow and Harlow, 1969 and 1970).

The results suggested that bodily contact (and not food) is the single most important requirement for the infant's attachment to its mother. Much more important, however, was the finding that 'monkeys which have known no affection can never develop either normal sexual behaviour or normal maternal behaviour and are bound to live out their lives as social failures'. This applied equally to male and female monkeys. Those females who did become pregnant – thanks to the persistence of normally-reared males – turned out to be 'hopeless, helpless and heartless mothers': either they ignored their babies or else they abused them brutally.

Studies with other animals, such as rats and goats, have produced similar results. These findings are striking enough to lend strong support to the hypothesis that being deprived of love and security in early life may well have similar long-term consequences in man; however, their exact nature must await the findings of further research.

Impaired family relationships

The importance of relationships to the child's optimal development has been implicit in much that has already been discussed. Here a closer look is taken at the long-term effects, when relations are severely or chronically disturbed, whether at home or in school.

The emotional climate of the home depends largely on the success of the parents' marriage, and temperamental, intellectual or sexual incompatibility often leads to a tense atmosphere, if not to open quarrels. Even when the child is not deliberately drawn into these, his own adjustment is likely to be affected. Similarly, if one parent is inadequate or mentally ill, it will affect not only the marital situation but also the parenting capacity of the affected partner (Quinton and Rutter, 1985).

A child from a discordant home is liable himself to become emotionally disturbed or antisocial, and not infrequently educationally backward too. A quarrelling, inadequate or disturbed parent makes a poor adult model. Evidence is now accumulating that parental hostility has a particularly harmful effect on a child's later development, especially on his ability to give as an adult unselfish loving care in the parental relationship. Thus parental hostility perpetuates itself from one generation to another in what is literally an extremely vicious circle.

Several studies both in this country and the USA show that parents who assault or otherwise injure their babies share a number of characteristics: the parents had been treated similarly themselves; even if they had not suffered quite the same violence, they had all been deprived of good mothering and been subjected to constant parental criticism. As adults they have quite unreasonably high expectations of their baby: his inability to conform with demands for obedience is seen as wilful and deliberate defiance; the baby's crying is interpreted as his refusal to love the parent; a punitive self-righteousness results in severe measures to 'discipline' him at a totally inappropriate age. Often too the battering parent is socially isolated and failing to find in the marriage partner the fulfilment of unmet needs (Hughes, 1967; Helfer and Kempe, 1968; Skinner and Castle, 1969; Jobling, 1977; Hyman, 1980).

Inevitably treatment of such a parent is both complex and lengthy. This poses extremely difficult issues. These are, at present, generally speaking, not being faced realistically; also they are considered more from the point of view of the battering parent than that of the infant, and his long-term welfare. Surely, the future safety of the injured child ought to be of paramount importance? Punishment of the parent helps neither him nor the child; yet returning the baby to a dangerous home where there is a high risk of further attack and injury, both physical and emotional, seems even less justifiable (Pringle, 1981).

Preoccupation with inter-personal stress and (for the child) insoluble conflict tend to interfere with successful learning. Also unsatisfactory relations with parents may make the establishment of good relations with other authority figures more difficult; this is likely to apply particularly to teachers in so far as the child perceives them to be *in loco parentis*.

> Parental mental disorder is most likely to be followed by behavioural disturbance in the children when the parent exhibits long-standing abnormalities of personality...The involvement of the child in the symptoms of the parental illness does seem to be crucial...Children in families where both parents are ill or where the parental illness is accompanied by break-up of the marriage seem to be especially at risk (Rutter, 1966).

Of course, genetic factors predisposing to mental illness in the adult may also play some part in the child's disturbance but available evidence suggests that this is not a major factor.

There is evidence too, that in homes where the father has been absent for long periods or permanently, boys are at greater risk of becoming delinquent and girls of having an illegitimate baby; but little is known as yet about the age at which absence is particularly harmful or relatively least damaging. The death of a parent appears to have a delayed or 'sleeper' effect: children bereaved in early childhood (but not infancy) seem most at risk but often emotional disturbance does not develop until adolescence. This is particularly so when the parent of the same sex has died, perhaps because this deprives the child of a model for adult behaviour as he reaches maturity (Rutter, 1966).

It looks as if there is a particularly close link between the home background, the child's educational achievements and antisocial behaviour (West, 1969; West and Farrington, 1977). In two long-term studies in which quite large groups of juvenile delinquents were followed up, respectively for eight and thirty years, it was found that seriously antisocial youngsters and especially recidivists showed these tendencies while still quite young; that a high proportion came from neglecting, disrupted and broken homes; that the majority had fathers who did semi-skilled or unskilled work; and that the children themselves had low ability and even lower educational achievements (Robins, 1966; Wolfgang et al., 1972).

Affection for and acceptance of children are not, of course, the prerogative of any social class; nor are impaired family relationships confined to any stratum of society. However, they may come to light more readily when a family is beset by social and economic problems, which come to the attention of the helping services. Since impaired relations are almost inevitably more frequent where there are such problems, children from socially and economically deprived homes are at greater risk.

They are also at greater risk educationally.

> Even in these latter days when so much has been written and so much is known about the causes of social and personal maladjustment, school often proves, for some unlucky youngster, to be a painful and sometimes a permanently damaging experience...Neither delinquency nor maladjustment are solely products of school life yet strain and tension induced by formal education could produce such results in children who are particularly stress-prone or who are already emotionally disturbed...How much misery is still inflicted upon children in school (and in their own homes, too, for that matter) it is quite impossible to estimate (Mays, 1974).

The major harm is probably done by teachers who undermine a child's confidence by constant disapproval and by irony; and who kill his joy in learning by dreary teaching, a permanent preoccupation with marks and rigid streaming, and by being interested in him only as a pupil rather than as an individual. Secondary schools are more likely to inflict such harm than primary schools, since, in the former, teaching is usually subject-orientated rather than child-centred.

THE NEED FOR NEW EXPERIENCES

Both under- and over-stimulation can have damaging effects, even on adults. One of the worst punishments is solitary confinement which deprives the individual of social interaction and severely restricts sensory and intellectual stimulation; even a monotonous or restricted environment is difficult to endure (as shown by polar expeditions as well as by research in the armed forces), producing depression, anxiety, irritability and a disruption of the ability to think clearly. Very similar consequences may well result from over-stimulation.

The exact difference which an enriching or depriving upbringing and home background can make, needs a great deal more research.

> However, a conservative estimate of the effect of extreme environments on intelligence is about 20 I.Q. points. This could mean the difference between a life in an institution for the subnormal or a productive life in society. It could mean the difference between a professional career and an occupation which is at the semi-skilled or unskilled level (Bloom, 1964).

Under-stimulation

The more uneventful and dull life is, the more readily boredom, frustration and restlessness set in. This is shown clearly by the contrast between the eagerness, alertness and vitality of normal toddlers whose life is filled with new experiences and challenges; and the aimlessness and boredom of adolescents with nothing to do and nowhere to go. The urban environment – in which the majority of the population now live – is hostile to the young; there is little freedom or safety to explore or experiment, particularly without adult supervision (Ward, 1978).

Too small houses or flats, small, formal gardens or playgrounds (if any) and dangerously busy roads severely restrict the space and freedom for unsupervised play. Conversely, children who are allowed to roam about freely, find themselves far too readily in conflict with the law through curiosity and a sense of adventure. Yet making adequate provision for both indoor and outdoor play and leisure facilities is still considered an unjustifiably costly 'frill'. Even adventure playgrounds, which in any case are few and far between, are fixed in location and duration as well as being circumscribed in providing scope for real discovery.

In seeking – legitimately – the excitement of new experiences where few are to be found or attainable, the forbidden, risky or dangerous are liable to acquire an aura of daring and excitement. What may start as a lark – an expression of high spirits and the desire for adventure – can all too readily turn into vandalism and other delinquency.

> It does not seem fanciful (though it remains to be proven) to suggest that some adolescent escapades which result in crime are child's play conducted with adult means, that the exaggerated need to identify with a group is a reaction to a depersonalised and incomplete experience of a human community...yet active challenge is comparatively rare, in spite of the attention it gets from the courts and the press; even juvenile delinquents amount to less than three per cent of the age group (Wall, 1968).

In the young child, insufficient sensory stimulation can retard or even impair development, including intellectual growth.

During recent years, the concept of infant intelligence has in fact assumed a new look. Marked individual differences have been observed quite early during the baby's first year of life and there is evidence that they are likely to be due to the effects of social stimulation (Kagan, 1971). If further studies confirm this, are remedial procedures required before the child has even left the cradle?

Probably the single and in the long run most crucial factor which promotes intellectual growth is the quality of the child's speech environment: not merely how much he is talked to, but how relevant, distinctive and rich the conversation is. The most essential element is the reciprocity of speech between child and adult, the latter initiating or responding to conversation. Hence, the mere presence of adults or just listening to conversation (on T.V. for example) is insufficient.

That this is so is shown by the comparatively more limited verbal ability of canal-boat and gypsy children as well as those reared in large families or those where language skills are very limited (Davie, Butler and Goldstein, 1972; Douglas 1964; Douglas, Ross and Simpson, 1968; Prosser, 1973; Rutter and Mittler, 1972). Such children have more contacts with other children than with adults; their language environment is less rich and possibly also less clear – because there is competing noise, whether from other children or the constantly switched on radio or television; and there is less likely to be an active enjoyment of language as a means of thought and communication. In consequence, the acquisition of verbal ability is adversely affected; this in turn affects the ability to respond to formal education, in particular to learning to read and write – the key skills to further scholastic progress.

Language has two main roles. It is a communication system – a way of sharing ideas and information with others; its second and probably more important role lies in controlling thought and, through it, behaviour. This is not to say that there can be no thought without language. Rather, thought remains markedly impoverished without language, perhaps in a real sense sub-human. Language is to thought what a catalyst is to a chemical reaction: it sets it off, speeds it up and facilitates it. Exactly how children learn to internalise language into thought remains to be explored in detail (Russia's A. R. Luria being one of the leaders of such studies); some linguists, it should be added, question the validity of these psychological theories.

Cultural and linguistic disadvantages

During the past ten years language development has grown to be a topic of central interest to educators, psychologists and sociologists; the concept of cultural and linguistic disadvantage, however, has become an issue of intense political controversy. In the fifties (and to some extent still now, *vide* Jensen, Taylor, Eysenck), theories of intelligence and intelligence testing were the focus of similar debates. The increasingly accepted current view is that tests are among the most useful tools for assessing a child's present level of functioning in the areas of performance for which the particular test has been designed – no more and no less; a minority continue to see them as an evil instrument of capitalistic or middle-class elitism and hence argue that they should be abolished.

It has been known for at least thirty years that children growing up in unstimulating environments – whether these be their own homes or institutions – often have limited language skills. But the sixties saw an upsurge of interest in linguistics and the birth of a new hypothesis, namely that language shapes not only thought but also (via various other processes) social class (Bernstein, 1961 and 1972). This goes much further, of course, than saying that language indicates social class. It postulates that the different language modes, characteristically used by the middle and the working classes, initiate and then reinforce different patterns of behaviour and personality. Thus they are held to perpetuate the structure of society itself. They have been respectively termed 'restricted' and 'elaborated' codes: the former is a stereotyped, condensed way of speaking, with short, simple and often incomplete sentences, generally rather limited in range and detail; whereas the middle-class language is held to be just the reverse. 'As the child learns his speech, so will he learn his social structure: and the latter will become the substratum of his innermost experience.'

Some American studies have reached similar conclusions. For example:

> Given these two kinds of communication networks within the family, repeated thousands of times in many different situations in the pre-school years, children from the two kinds of families can hardly fail to enter school with quite different capabilities for receiving and processing information...for defining the world, understanding it, or developing strategies for ordering it (Hess and Shipman, 1965).

Also the ability to motivate children to be attentive is important in developing intellectual capabilities to the full (Stinchcombe, 1969). If these views are accepted, they would seem to provide the answer to the question which has increasingly exercised educators: why do so many working-class children fail in school despite the fact that the British educational system has become increasingly open?

There is a four-way and largely ideological split about how to solve this problem. First, the politically committed, radical spokesman argues that these views on the role of language serve to protect the privileges and power of the ruling middle-class elite, particularly within the educational system. Moreover, he is highly critical of the theory itself on a number of grounds; these include that far too little is known about working-class language and its relationship to class, Bernstein and others notwithstanding; that the research methodology of recorded interviews with mothers itself militates against obtaining the richness of the vernacular culture of the street, resulting instead in atypical inarticulate responses; that the influences of other powerful agencies of socialisation, besides the home, school and peer group, are being ignored, from the mass media to non-conformist chapels and brass bands; and that much of middle-class speech is anyhow turgid, redundant, empty and lacking in vitality (Baratz and Baratz, 1970; Barnes, Britton and Rosen, 1971; Labov, 1971).

Secondly, some educational reformers, who believe in working from within the system, refute the accusation that teachers are aiming to impose middle-class values on working-class children; in any case, they believe that middle-class values encompass two different systems, one of status-striving and the other based on intellectual interests: often they go together since academic achievements are among the main means for improving status, but there is no inevitable or intrinsic link between them.

Instead, they argue that the teacher's task is to widen the horizons of the children whose homes are insufficiently stimulating and to initiate them into more subtle and complex ways of thinking and reasoning. The aim is to free them from the mental confines of their environment and to extend their range of values – which they may or may not accept subsequently. They hold that to preserve the social status quo or to introduce a kind of educational apartheid with popular education based on the folk culture of the working class would mean insulating class cultures from each other; either aim serves to dampen down working-class aspirations to an intellectually and materially richer life which compensatory education seeks to encourage.

Thirdly, the progressive humanist and environmentalist sees compensatory education as a means of overcoming 'cultural', 'social' or 'linguistic' disadvantage or deprivation; the earlier it is provided and the more the family, and in particular the mother, can be involved, the more likely it is to be successful. Fourthly, the conservative and reactionary believer in heredity uses impoverished language development as the justification for maintaining two separate systems of education, one rigorously academic, the other vocational and practical.

Bernstein himself (1971) seems to be speaking with two voices, as is demonstrated by the following quotations from the same book:

> the normal linguistic environment of the working class is one of linguistic deprivation [page 66];...The concept of 'compensatory education' implies that something is lacking in the family, and so in the child...the school has to 'compensate' for the something which is missing...and the children become little deficit systems...Once the problem is seen even implicitly in this way, then it becomes appropriate to coin the terms 'cultural deprivation', 'linguistic deprivation', etc. and then these labels do their sad work [page 192].

Confusion becomes worse confounded when Bernstein's use of the term 'working class' is examined. On the one hand, he says his concept of linguistic deprivation applies only to the unskilled working class, but on the other he claims that these constitute 29 per cent of the population. Yet according to the Registrar General's classification of occupations, unskilled workers comprise 8 per cent and semi-skilled 20 per cent of the population. Nor are all, or even the majority, of children from unskilled working-class homes either linguistically or educationally deprived by any definition.

This was again shown by the results of the *National Child Development Study* (Davie, Butler and Goldstein, 1972): regarding oral ability some 40 per cent, and in reading attainment some 48 per cent, of children whose fathers are unskilled were said by their teachers to be below the average (and 10 per cent and 7 per cent respectively markedly poor); the proportions were somewhat lower for children whose fathers are semi-skilled. In other words, Bernstein's conclusions would seem to apply at most to some 10 per cent rather than almost 30 per cent of the population. Nor are such learning difficulties confined to any one class; even in Social Class I and II, some 15 per cent of the children were found to have below average oral and some 13 per cent below average reading ability (but only about 2 per cent were markedly poor).

In my view, insufficient intellectual and language stimulation is as real a problem as under-nourishment used to be. And, in a similar way, such mental under-nourishment is likely to be the result of an unfavourable total environment – poor housing, low income, poorer physical care, an unstable family structure and a culturally impoverished home leading to intellectual malnutrition.

On the one hand, the consequences of such complex and interacting patterns of disadvantage cannot be remedied by the school alone; on the other hand, many secondary schools compound the damage by their subject-centred organisation which makes for minimal personal interaction between teacher and pupil, and by a curriculum which too often has little relevance to their interests or future lives.

With regard to American 'enrichment' or 'compensatory' programmes, they were launched with too high hopes (also they were often too 'symptom specific'). Now they are being dismissed with similarly unwarranted disappointment. It was unrealistic to expect a few extra hours of schooling, available for a year or two, together with a few excursions to tip the scales against such powerful factors as poverty, ignorance, disease and despair, to which the children had been exposed for years and in which they continued to live.

These special programmes did not succeed in enabling disadvantaged children to catch up in those academic skills which can be measured, in particular in respect of intelligence quotients which often were the sole criterion used. Nevertheless, as the massive Coleman report (1966) and later research conclude, there were considerable gains. Indeed, any broadening experience must be counted as a net gain.

The urban aid and educational priority areas programmes in the UK appear to have made somewhat greater impact but it is too early to judge their long-term effectiveness in stimulating intellectual and language development (Halsey, 1972; Mortimore and Blackstone, 1982). A real breakthrough will require a multi-pronged and sustained approach, including parental support and involvement; even then, dramatic or quick changes are highly unlikely (Pilling and Pringle, 1978).

Over-stimulation

In the young child, over-stimulation may lead to uncontrollable excitement, tenseness, exhaustion and disturbed sleep. In the adult, too, the ability to cope may become impaired if he has to grapple with unfamiliar or unpredictable events, relationships or objects at too great a pace. This is shown, for example, by the traveller who suffers from 'culture shock' when plunged into an alien environment without adequate preparation. The need to adapt rapidly and repeatedly to changing conditions produces disorientation and distortion of reality, anxiety or extreme irritability; eventually fatigue, apathy and withdrawal may set in.

Sensory bombardment can have as devastating effects as deprivation (and is used for similar purposes in political brain-washing). In the early months of life, one of the functions of good mothering is to act as a filter or barrier to avoid over-stimulation; yet later on some young people seem to seek a surfeit of sound and movement in discotheques, perhaps because there is not enough stimulation in their everyday life.

Similarly, on the cognitive and decision-making level, attention wanders and performance deteriorates at school or at work, when there is insufficient challenge; yet if there is too much to learn or understand – or if in the factory the conveyor belt moves too fast – then confusion, mistakes, tenseness and frustration result. Research has shown that, whatever the task, there is for each individual an optimal level of stimulation and a marked excess leads to stress and maladaptation (Miller, 1964; Sargeant, 1963; Selye, 1978).

Recently the thesis has been put forward that contemporary society is plunging headlong into accelerating and unmanageable change; and that unless measures are taken to prepare the young – and the community at large – to cope with it, a condition termed 'future shock' will result (Toffler, 1973). This is defined as 'the distress, both physical and psychological, that arises from overload of the human organism's physical adaptive systems and its decision-making processes . . . it is the human response to over-stimulation'.

Arguing that ours is becoming a 'throw-away society' in which things, people and organisational forms are becoming disposable, Toffler suggests that children are being trained from early on for 'turn-over and disaffiliation', due to frequently moving home and losing friends, and to the high rate of turnover among teachers. At the same time, 'our time perspective on education is unbalanced. At school we go heavily into the past, minimally into the present and zero into the future'. The accelerating rate of change is enforcing a new life pace where mastery of new situations becomes essential in ever shorter intervals. For some this 'overload' leads to confusional breakdown; signs of this, in Toffler's view, are the spreading use of tranquillisers and drugs; the rise of mysticism; the revolt of the young; the recurrent outbreaks of violence and vandalism; and the politics of nihilism and anarchy.

The so-called 'rat-race' probably plays a major part in the alienation and opting-out of the young from apparently 'good' middle-class homes. Pressurised by status and achievement-orientated parents towards what is seen by them as success without being given much of their parents' time or indeed affection; with few other values or ideals being put before them, either at home or at (usually boarding) schools; is it surprising that such young people prefer a future different from that mapped out by their parents?

When we consider together the urge of youth to rebel – to escape, to be adventurous – and the current openings for unconventional life-styles, what is remarkable is how strong the pull towards conformity remains. The picture of youth as in total revolt is a quite false presentation. For every out-and-out rebel, whether of the blatantly destructive or of the intelligently critical kind, there are many others in the same age-range and situation who accept without question the expectations of those in authority... The number of conformist adolescents puts in question the popular assumption of an exceptional 'generation gap' today. That such a gap exists between some young people and some adults is obvious. Communication may break down completely. But in other families the communication and cooperation are of a frankness and friendliness which seem to be far in advance of the norms of 1910, or even 1930, when, for the most part, no communication between the generations on personal matters was expected, and the role accorded to young people was not to discuss but to obey (Hemming, 1974).

THE NEED FOR PRAISE AND RECOGNITION

Unfortunately, praise and recognition are almost invariably given for achievement and not for effort. In consequence, this need is most readily and often satisfied in the case of intelligent, healthy, adjusted and attractive children (who are even praised merely for their pleasing appearance!).

In contrast, the intellectually slow, the culturally disadvantaged, the emotionally neglected or disturbed get far less, if any, praise and recognition. Yet their need is very much greater. Whatever small successes they achieve inevitably demand far more effort and perseverance; yet they receive less reward because they achieve less. Worse still, those who are rejected by their parents, and regarded as failures by their teachers, are wholly deprived of the satisfaction of this need by adults.

Even ability and talent well above the average may never declare themselves if adequate nurture or emotional support is lacking. The quality of family relationships, the emotional climate of the home, together with parental interest and encouragement, are of paramount importance also in helping able children to realise their potential (Pringle, 1970). Reviewing the causes of failure among gifted children, Burt (1975) concluded: 'Many of the parents appeared entirely indifferent to the child's success either in school or even in later life'.

Of course, no environment guarantees high achievement or consigns children irrevocably to low achievement. But a much higher proportion with unrealised potential will be found among certain economic sectors, social classes, ethnic groups and geographic areas than in others. Recent years have seen a conflict of viewpoint between those who argue that everyone must be given an equal educational opportunity and those who advocate that special attention ought to be devoted to the abler child. The former make a case for positive discrimination in favour of the socially and culturally disadvantaged child; whereas the latter claim that a country's ability to compete successfully in a scientific and technological age depends on the fostering of excellence.

The conflict between these two standpoints is, however, more apparent than real. It springs from the mistaken belief that all men are equal despite the enormous disparity found in physical and intellectual potential in all walks of life. To be given equality of opportunity is the right of every child; to expect equal capacity to make use of this opportunity runs counter to common sense and experience. Indeed, it has harmful consequences because such expectation is bound to engender a sense of failure.

Instead, we must act as if all children were equal and then respect, as well as accept and cater for, their differences. This means giving recognition to and developing all the different abilities and talents a child may have. Within such a framework, it is legitimate both to provide a democracy of opportunity while at the same time to strive for excellence so as to ensure an aristocracy of achievement.

Can the need for praise and recognition be 'over-satisfied', as it were? There seem to be two different ways in which this may happen. First, when praise and recognition are given too readily, then the child will not be encouraged to give of his best but be satisfied with the results of too limited an effort; or he may ignore such undeserved praise altogether because it has become devalued in his eyes, so that once again it will be ineffective as an incentive.

Secondly, when parents make achievement almost a condition of their love, then this may lead to the development in the child of an abnormally strong drive for success, esteem and power. Perhaps this is the driving force behind some of the strikingly successful people in business, sport or the arts, who seem to be spurred on by an almost insatiable need for praise and recognition which to them probably spells 'love'.

If this need is inadequately met or remains unsatisfied, then in the long term the effects are destructive of self-respect and of confidence in tackling new situations, tasks or relationships.

The role of competition

Another and linked difficulty relates to the belief – which is probably based on our puritan tradition – that the spur of competition leads to greatly increased effort; in this context, even the idea that all children must experience a measure of success is suspect. In fact, one of the most difficult challenges to parents and teachers is how, despite differences both in ability and in emotional development, all children can be helped to achieve some success.

The intensely competitive climate of our society, which is mirrored in the family and in the educational system, gives rise to two difficulties. First, if all children had equal ability and opportunities, then competition would be a measure of effort made. Because they have not, the same group remains comparatively unsuccessful. (The belief that the intellectually or verbally less competent are better with their hands is not corroborated by evidence.)

If a goal is felt to be unattainable, effort diminishes, partly because the cumulative effect of failure leads to a sense of hopelessness and partly because feeling rejected as being 'no good' arouses anxiety which further inhibits learning. Under-achievement, like envy, seems to feed on itself. A poor start in school snowballs into chronic failure and the teacher's understandable disappointment with poor progress only serves to lead to further discouragement in the pupil. And so both are caught in the vicious circle of discouragement, disapproval, unresponsiveness and further failure. The more competitive the system, the greater the proportion of children who are doomed to failure since only a select few can succeed. Moreover, an emphasis on competition tends to lead to an emotional climate where winning becomes the most important goal; learning for its own sake takes a back seat.

The second difficulty lies in the fact that an emphasis on competition interferes with the development of cooperative attitudes. Both experimental and clinical studies have demonstrated the disruptive effects of competition. If cooperative behaviour has survival value, then the skills of cooperation are far more basic to successful living than those of competition. Yet many children are exposed by their parents to a very competitive climate, siblings and other children being held up to them as examples, even when emulation is beyond the child's capacity. Similarly, parental expectations and pressures bear a measure of responsibility for the competitive atmosphere which prevails in many schools. (After all, some mothers start being competitive by comparing their babies' bladder control!)

Undoubtedly, children themselves create many competitive situations and test their abilities in countless ways of their own; these provide a means of realising their strength and discovering their limitations. When the yardstick is his own previous level of performance, maturation and experience alone will assure success; adding the incentive of recognition and encouraging the child to aim at surpassing his own past achievement are the surest road to progress and to establishing his self-esteem. These will then in turn act as powerful incentives to further effort.

How effective is group work compared with individual work? A lot of research has been done on this aspect of teaching and the general conclusion is that individual work is more fruitful when dealing with simple techniques where there is nothing to be gained from an exchange of views.

But there is general agreement that more advanced intellectual operations benefit from group work. This seems to be because more suggestions are put forward; the quality of the work tends to be set by the level of the most able members of the group; since they will be judged by their peers, the individuals are keen to cooperate and to show up well; ideas proposed are subjected to immediate approval or criticism (Hotyat, 1974).

The teacher's role

Because the school is more overtly concerned with standards of attainment and assessment of performance than the home, success and failure inevitably assume a major role. Streaming, marks and examinations are all means of publicly, as it were, recognising achievement or the lack of it. What has just been said about the role of competition applies with even greater force to the class-room: it is primarily achievement which calls forth recognition, the more so the older the child; and because the teacher is in a much better position than the parent to view a child's performance in relation to that of his contemporaries, disapproval and failure acquire an additional dimension.

Yet praising for achievement instead of effort has very harmful effects on the slower learner as well as on the child with emotional or physical handicaps: he has no chance of shining and always finds himself near the bottom. Such constant failure inevitably damages self-esteem and motivation. Nor do able children benefit from a highly competitive school regime, because they can do better than average without necessarily giving of their best or even trying very hard; this tends to breed arrogance and complacency, neither of which are conducive to effort or a spirit of cooperation. The teacher who believes that what matters most is the effort a child makes, and who praises whenever there is progress, however slow and limited, provides an appropriate incentive for all pupils, whatever their abilities.

The recent evidence that the foundation for intellectual and emotional growth is laid long before the start of compulsory schooling might have a rather depressing effect on teachers. They might reason that if parental attitudes to education are so vital to the child's response to education, if home circumstances outweigh the effect of schooling, then what hope is there that schools can bring about any radical improvement? Such a defeatist attitude on the part of the teacher would inevitably be transmitted to a pupil without its being spelt out; in turn it would affect his own attitude and hence his level of progress, as much if not more than his actual ability.

However, some even more recent research justifies a much more optimistic attitude on two grounds: it has shown just how potent are parental participation on the one hand, and the expectations of teachers on the other in influencing children's progress (Meyers, 1973; Pidgeon 1970; Rutter et al., 1979; Wall 1973; Wiseman 1972). One example must suffice. Pupils with similar attainment levels were given intelligence tests and then their teachers were told that some had better learning potential than expected, whereas others were slow learners. A follow-up examination showed that those pupils, who the teachers had been led to expect could do better, were in fact doing better than the others, although the two groups had been matched for ability at the outset (Rosenthal and Jacobsen, 1968).

This finding underlines the truth of the saying 'give a dog a bad name'; labelling a child 'slow' (or 'bright') becomes a self-fulfilling prophecy. And this is as powerful in affecting the teacher (and parent) as it is in affecting how the child feels about himself, whether he thinks he is stupid or capable, and how hard he tries: self-confidence and motivation are fostered or extinguished by the way teachers think about and treat their charges.

Work experience

When a young person starts work, he is once again in a situation in which his self-respect may become enhanced or diminished. In our competitive society, exams and certificates have practically become the hall-mark of success; not only for climbing up the economic ladder but even for finding employment when the need for unskilled labour is contracting. Hence for those who have done badly in the educational system, the chances are high that they will only be able to obtain jobs which carry the lowest level of recognition in terms of both prestige and pay. Technical advances, together with automation, are making even undemanding jobs scarce so that opportunities for unskilled teenagers have greatly diminished. Also the less able, educationally backward school leaver is particularly hard hit by a high level of unemployment.

Enforced idleness, boredom and little money in his pocket tend to undermine further what limited self-respect is left to the adolescent who has for years been caught in a web of multiple disadvantages, including being denied the satisfaction and spur of praise and recognition. Feeling that society disowns him may well engender a feeling that he in turn owes nothing to society.

THE NEED FOR RESPONSIBILITY

Society is ambiguous and ambivalent about granting responsibility and independence, particularly during adolescence. This is reflected in the way in which various adult rights – such as to enter a public house, to consume alcohol, to drive a car, to vote, to work part- or full-time, to marry without parental consent – are conceded at different ages. Parents and teachers differ even more widely in the amount of independence they are prepared to allow or to tolerate and in the extent to which they expect responsible behaviour without at the same time granting the right to make responsible decisions.

To thrust too much responsibility onto a child or to do so too early may have harmful effects. Without the necessary understanding of what is involved and of the probable consequences of a particular decision or choice, responsibility will be perceived as a burden. He may nevertheless be prepared to shoulder it but at a high cost in terms of anxiety; or he may refuse to accept it, spending much time and ingenuity in devising ways of avoiding responsibility, perhaps wishing and dreaming but rarely doing.

The child who is denied opportunities to exercise responsibility will fail to develop a sense of responsibility for himself, for others or for material objects. When this denial has gone hand in hand with a lack of training in self-control and in planning ahead, then such youngsters will tend to be impulsive, unwilling to postpone immediate gratification of impulses, and contemptuous of the rights of others – in short, irresponsible.

It is likely that the self-same youngsters will later on find themselves in jobs which give them little, if any, responsibility. Work which fails to fulfil the need for involvement is likely to heighten the sense of alienation and irresponsibility which is bred by being made to feel an educational and vocational reject. Work which is repetitive, undemanding and frequently carried on in noisy or otherwise unpleasant conditions, is likely to induce both boredom and frustration. Whether at school or at work, these probably account for the craving of so many young people to find, in their spare time, excitement and an outlet for bottled-up needs and energies.

Practice in decision-making

The freedom to make decisions is part of exercising responsibility. The steadily lengthening process of compulsory education means that young people remain financially dependent on their parents longer and dependent on their teachers in relation to a major part of their waking day. Yet as soon as they leave school, young people are faced today with a wide variety of choices and decisions. There is a bewildering range of jobs, of life-styles and of religious, political and social beliefs. Choices are particularly difficult and complex in two areas which involve the deepest and most personal feelings.

First, most adolescents are trying to grapple with questions relating to their eventual social and sexual adjustment in the adult world. Secondly, they are searching for some interpretation of life, however vague or tentatively formulated - perhaps no more than a *modus vivendi*, 'do as you would be done by' or some simple code of fair play – which would give some meaning and direction to their own behaviour and to that of others.

For many, little guidance is available either in their homes or at school. Perhaps this is because there is now a lack of certainty, of moral imperatives, of ready answers and traditional religious beliefs.

In this situation, it is tempting to evade the issues altogether. May it be that this evasion creates its own problems? Determined not to inculcate values, we instead almost avoid discussing them altogether, thus providing no reference points for the many decisions later demanded by life itself? Is it because we have failed to provide appropriate nourishment for the imagination of many young people, and adequate support in their search for meaning, that they are seeking it in the hallucinations of drugs or are opting out altogether? Or because they feel the standards of the previous generation to be irrelevant or even immoral in the context of today? It is vital for youngsters to consider 'preferable futures'. Some may at present spend ten or more years in school without ever being encouraged to look at their value-systems and to ask themselves: 'What kind of life do I want to lead?' or 'What kind of person do I want to become?'

Preparation for parenthood

A strong case could be made out for including three new areas of knowledge in the curriculum of all secondary schools: first, an understanding of human psychology; second, preparation for parenthood; and thirdly, education for leisure. A knowledge of human psychology would include the dynamics of human conduct, the roots of prejudice and the ways in which people interact at a great variety of levels. This might contribute to an understanding or consciousness of one's self which is different from self-consciousness. Though difficult to acquire, it is probably more important than sex education or a knowledge of how the body functions; yet in practice it receives far less, if any, attention. Of course, schools alone cannot in any case be expected to bring this about.

To be effective, a programme of preparation for parenthood would have to adopt a wide base. 'Education' is too narrow a connotation, suggesting classes and instruction on the model of sex education; also, it conveys too formal a framework and too intellectual a conception, suggesting that 'knowing' is enough. What is required is neither a narrow course, seen as a branch of biology or home economics, nor a very wide, general one in citizenship; equally, it should not be confined, as it tends to be at present, to girls and the less able ones at that. Some first-hand experience of babies and young children should form an integral part of such a scheme.

The core of a course of preparation for parenthood should be an understanding of human psychology. This would not only offer a unifying theme but the focus and starting point would be the adolescents themselves. Their interest and involvement would readily be enlisted since at this stage of growth, intense but confused feelings and doubts about personal relationships are a normal preoccupation of young people. Thus an opportunity would be provided for them to acquire an understanding of the sequential nature of human development, of the various stages of physical and mental growth, of motivation and of the wide variations in behaviour, including deviancy.

Clearly this knowledge could be presented at differing levels of sophistication and depth according to the pupils' level of ability. It would be designed to complement and supplement what children will have learnt already in their own families. Teachers, however, can present such knowledge in a more systematic, more generalised and less personal way.

Included too should be an appreciation both of parental rights and responsibilities. At present, the father's role is rarely mentioned, while home-making and motherhood are undervalued. So much so that the housewife with small children, whose working hours are often twice as long as that of the thirty-five-hour-a-week clerk, is described and treated as not being gainfully employed.

Education for leisure is going to be an important part of education so long as the present unemployment situation remains as it is. In some areas of Britain employment opportunities are so scarce that work is the exception rather than the rule. Even for those in work, dull repetitive jobs are the norm. Education that allows for a surplus of leisure time and opens up ideas for creative pursuits will be very valuable. Until and unless available employment opportunities improve and working conditions become more satisfactory, parenting and leisure pursuits are likely to provide the major source of personal fulfilment. Shorter working hours are already on the way with increasing technological advances, particularly automation (Pringle, 1980).

Again, courses should be widely based, covering the many possible forms of physical recreation as well as an appreciation of what they can offer by way of a healthy mind in a healthy body. Also crafts of various kinds and in particular the cultivation of an appreciation of the arts and, better still, the confidence to participate creatively in at least one of them – can make a vital contribution to the development of emotional maturity and to the growth of a compassionate understanding of man's predicament. Giving young people the basis for an enjoyable use of leisure may, moreover, make it more likely that later on they will be prepared to seek opportunities for further education. If their memories of secondary education are happy, then one important step towards lifelong education – considered by many to be a necessary goal in a rapidly changing society – will have been taken, namely preventing a reluctance to go on learning (Wall, 1977; Whitfield, 1980).

Will-power or determinism

If the basic psychological needs remain unfulfilled, is a child doomed forever? And if he is not, what determines whether or not he succeeds in overcoming the ill-effects of early and cumulative deprivation? At present, no precise answers are available but opinions cover the whole range from determinism to the belief that everyone, given the will, can 'win through'.

Advocates of determinism run the risk of conveying to young people that a deprived early life is an excuse, indeed almost a justification, for subsequent violent, lawless or otherwise deviant behaviour. This belief is unwarrantably defeatist. Advocates of will-power are, however, unwarrantably optimistic since no one is entirely 'master of his fate', least of all those who – even from before birth – have been beset by a pattern of complex and continuing disadvantage.

The truth lies somewhere between these two extreme positions. In practice, we cannot but act as if it were never too late, as if rehabilitation and treatment always have a chance of success. Unless we do so, we shall not improve upon available methods. Even more important, applying therapeutic and remedial measures without real confidence in them is the surest recipe for failure.

6. Children Who Are 'Vulnerable' or 'At Risk'

The myth of childhood being a carefree, happy time persists despite scant evidence to substantiate it. On the contrary, there is much that frustrates, frightens and baffles the growing child just because of his inevitable lack of experience and power. The younger he is, the more he lives solely in the present and his time perspective is limited so that he does not even have the consolation that anxieties and unhappiness will pass. Nor does he know that his frequent feelings of uncertainty, his lack of confidence and his failure to understand adults' reactions, are shared by many, if not most, of his contemporaries. This awareness comes largely with maturity except for the fortunate minority whose parents and teachers have the gift of remembering these feelings and, by using their memories, enable the young to cope with them more easily.

In one sense, then, all children are vulnerable and likely to experience unhappiness and stress. In addition, certain groups are made doubly vulnerable because of the presence of specific, potentially detrimental personal, family or social circumstances. It is such children who should be regarded as being 'at risk'. The idea that certain individuals or groups may be at high risk of future misfortune or malfunctioning has for long been accepted and acted upon in the world of life or accident insurance. The concept of being 'at risk' psychologically, educationally or socially is beginning to gain currency, following its successful application in the medical field.

The Perinatal Survey (Butler and Bonham, 1963; Butler and Alberman, 1969), emphasised the danger signs which place a baby at high risk of dying. These were shown to be not only abnormalities of pregnancy and complications of labour, but also biological factors, such as extremes of maternal age, and social circumstances, such as low socio-economic status. Moreover, adverse social and biological characteristics tended to reinforce one another. There is evidence too that an unfavourable socio-economic environment continues to exert an adverse effect on the growing child. That this is so, at least until the age of eleven years, has been shown by the *National Child Development Study*. (National Children's Bureau, 1972).

To ensure the earliest diagnosis of defects, local health authorities were encouraged to keep 'at risk' registers of those babies thought to be vulnerable because of adverse circumstances before, during or after birth. Though some doubt has recently been cast on their effectiveness, there is evidence that they can be of considerable value (Davie, Butler and Goldstein, 1972); this is particularly so if it leads to the differential allocation of resources between 'high' and 'low' risk children – in other words, positive discrimination in favour of the most vulnerable.

Whether it is either desirable or practicable (or both) to keep a register of children who are psychologically, educationally or socially at risk is a controversial question. Undoubtedly, such a suggestion is fraught with difficulties, not least because of its political implications. Also knowledge regarding likely physical consequences is much better established than the understanding of psychological concomitants.

In essence, the issue is this: if later malfunctioning or handicap can be predicted early with a satisfactory degree of probability, then three consequences could follow as a matter of practical politics: first, to assess, and where necessary to refine, methods for identifying 'vulnerable' or 'at risk' groups at the earliest possible time; secondly, to devise procedures to prevent the harmful effects altogether if possible, or else to mitigate their severity; and thirdly, to evaluate the short- and long-term effectiveness of any interventionist procedures.

There are five groups of children who are particularly 'vulnerable' or 'at risk' of becoming stunted or damaged in their psychological development because of personal, family or social circumstances. They are: children in large families with low incomes; children with physical or mental handicaps; those in one-parent families; children who have to live apart from their parents for longer or shorter periods; and those belonging to some minority groups. There are, of course, other stressful circumstances such as living in a home where there is a chronically sick or disabled parent or a step-parent; or where the father is unemployed or follows a criminal career, spending long periods in prison; or where the child has been in a natural disaster. However, these five groups have been chosen because they include the great majority of children 'at risk'.

The various kinds of potentially harmful circumstances are not, of course, mutually exclusive. The exact proportion of children affected by one or more of them is not known. It could well be as high as 15 or 20 per cent but the proportion depends to some extent on the definitions and borderlines which are chosen.

It must also be stressed that none of these circumstances inevitably leads to psychological damage. To some extent, the concept of vulnerability is a statistical one, being rather like an actuarial prediction: it is concerned with likelihood, not certainty, in respect of any individual child. Indeed, there are many who triumph, apparently unscathed, over severe and prolonged environmental handicaps (Rutter and Madge, 1977).

LARGE FAMILIES WITH LOW INCOMES

In Great Britain at least three million children – or nearly a quarter of the child population under the age of fifteen years – are growing up in families of four or more children. As a group, they tend to be on average, relatively under-privileged whatever the socio-economic level of their parents. Some of the likely reasons for this have already been considered (see Chapter 3, page 66) but here we are concerned with families of limited means.

Some of the measurable effects

The most recent evidence from the *NCDS* demonstrates that the handicapping effects begin before birth and affect subsequent physical, psychological and educational development. This was so at the age of 7, 11 and 16 years (Davie, 1972; Prosser, 1973; Wedge and Prosser, 1973; Butler and Goldstein, 1973; Fogelman and Goldstein, 1976; Essen and Wedge, 1982).

Family size was found to have an adverse effect on both height and educational attainment. For example, the difference between a child who has no older siblings and one who has three or more was 2.8 cm height and fifteen months of reading attainment at the age of seven years. By the age of eleven years the difference had increased to 4.0 cm for height and twenty-nine months for reading. These findings applied irrespective of the father's occupation, the mother's height or the number of younger children in the family. It used to be thought that children's social adjustment in school was better when they came from large than from small families; more recent evidence, including the above study, has shown the opposite to be the case.

Children from large families with low incomes may also be at greater risk right from conception onwards because of their mother's smoking habits. It is now widely accepted that maternal smoking during pregnancy is associated with both a reduction in birthweight and an increase in perinatal mortality. In the *National Child Development Study* a higher proportion of mothers from working-class homes were smoking during pregnancy and, irrespective of social class, more mothers with large families (three or more children) were doing so while pregnant. After allowing for these factors, this had a measurable effect both on height and on educational attainment. Its size was the same at the age of seven and eleven years, namely 1.0 cm and four months in reading (Butler and Goldstein, 1973).

There are likely to be additional disadvantages since large families tend to occur more often in the lowest socio-economic groups. For example, in the *National Child Development Study* 5½ per cent of children in Social Class I and 32 per cent in Social Class V came from families with five or more children. Irrespective of family size, the income of semi- and unskilled workers is substantially lower than that of the other socio-economic groups (Central Statistical Office, 1986). Hence financial hardship is virtually inevitable despite various allowances and benefits where there is a large family. According to official figures, 4 out of 10 large families were living on low incomes (defined as up to 140 per cent of supplementary benefit level); and of all families where the father was in work, 11 per cent were living on low incomes (Child Poverty Action Group, 1984).

The disadvantages of belonging to a large, low income family are further magnified by the consequences of suffering from other associated shortcomings. The parents' own education, parental interest shown in the child's scholastic progress, housing, play space, household amenities such as indoor sanitation or running hot water – all these and many other circumstances are more frequently unfavourable in such homes. Furthermore, a whole range of adverse factors is often found together so that the resulting consequences on the child's development are in most cases both multiple and interrelated.

Some results from the Bureau's longitudinal study will illustrate this interlinked pattern of continuing and cumulative disadvantage. When both the father and mother stayed on at school beyond the minimum school-leaving age, they were likely to have a smaller family; also they were more likely to show a greater interest in their children's education (at the age of eleven years). In turn, both parental education and parental interest were, separately and measurably, associated with the children's actual level of scholastic attainment – the effect of each being the equivalent of, for instance, almost a year's reading age and a combined effect of nineteen months at the age of seven years.

At this early age, the overall effect of social disadvantage, and hence readiness to respond to educational expectations, is already clearly evident. After two years of schooling, the chance of a seven-year-old's being unable to read was fifteen times greater for a child from an unskilled working-class home (Social Class V) than from a professional (Social Class I); and the proportion of children from the former who would – in the opinion of their teachers – benefit from attending a special school was forty-five times larger than for those from a professional home.

Another example relates to housing. To begin with, there is a relationship between family size and over-crowding: the larger the former, the worse the incidence of the latter is likely to be. Thus whereas 57 per cent of children from families with five or more children were over-crowded, the incidence fell to only 4 per cent where there were not more than four children. Over-crowding remained a problem, so that by the age of eleven (i.e., in 1969), as many as one in eight of this nationally representative group lived in such conditions. Next, there was a very marked social class difference: children from unskilled working-class homes were ten times more likely to live in an over-crowded home than those from professional-class parents. Thirdly, the larger the number of children the less likely the family was to enjoy the sole use of such amenities as a bathroom, indoor lavatory and hot water supply.

Clearly stress and hardship are further magnified the larger the number of children. Cramped conditions which deny privacy, space for play and quiet for homework readily lead to irritability, restlessness and bad temper all round. Inevitably the brunt of the burden is carried by the mother who is rearing a family without the basic amenities which are taken for granted by the more fortunate majority.

These problems are further aggravated because outdoor play space is at a premium in practically all urban areas. The poverty of recreational provision is indicated by the fact that nearly three times as many mothers expressed dissatisfaction with available amenities as were dissatisfied with housing conditions (33 per cent compared with 12 per cent); a government study has corroborated our findings (Department of the Environment, 1973). This situation is likely to be worse for children living in deprived city areas where houses and flats are commonly without a private garden or yard.

Again, over-crowding and a lack of amenities had considerable and measurable effects on educational attainment, social adjustment and health. For example, at the age of eleven years, over-crowding was associated with a retardation of about seventeen months in reading age and of twelve months where amenities were lacking – a combined effect of almost two and a half years. This is more marked than the effects had been at the age of seven years (nine months' retardation in relation to over-crowding and nine months also in relation to amenities).

Taken together these findings point to three conclusions. First, many children growing up in large families whose income is low, are beset by multiple, interrelated and interacting disadvantages which have a detrimental effect on the level of their educational attainment, social adjustment in school and probably also on their physical development, in particular height. Secondly, these effects usually work in combination and are cumulative. Thirdly, their adverse influence seems to increase over time so that the gap between the most advantaged and the most disadvantaged grows wider as the child grows older.

At least, this is the case in the Bureau's longitudinal study; for example, the combined effect of social disadvantage on reading attainment showed itself in a 4-year gap at the age of 7 (a good reader having attained the level of an average 9-year-old while 5 years is usually taken as the level of a non-reader). By the time the children were 11 years old, it had risen to a difference of 8 years between the most advantaged and disadvantaged respectively (Davie, 1973; N.C.B., 1972), and differences persisted into the teens (Fogelman, 1983).

This finding of a widening gap in reading attainment during the junior school years confirms the results of an earlier study (Douglas,

1964). It also reinforces the view that equality of opportunity will not come about through changes in secondary or higher education. Rather it is during the pre-school and early school years that ways must be sought to overcome or compensate for the consequences of environmental disadvantages on children's development. Limiting the initial gap is likely to be the most effective way of reducing the gap at later stages (Fogelman and Gorbach, 1978; Russell, 1979).

Effects on family relationships and on personal development

There is a tendency to paint a rather rosy picture of lower working-class life, according to which mutual self-help and support in child rearing, as well as in general family and financial matters, play a major part. It is doubtful whether this is in fact the dominant pattern in areas of high social need. In reality, more often than not, all members of the extended family in deprived urban neighbourhoods suffer from multiple disadvantages which stem from low income, poor housing and a limited ability to cope. Poor health and irregular employment not infrequently add to the difficulties.

For those at the lowest rung of the social and economic ladder, even collective resources have little to offer. Shared misery may temporarily lighten the weight of the burden but it is unlikely either to reduce its effect materially or to alleviate its causes. Grandparents may add another dimension to children's lives by providing a three-generation perspective; yet they also make heavy inroads on very limited family budgets. Other relations may contribute some cast-off clothes or a little cash in times of financial crisis, but usually they can do little to improve grossly inadequate housing or income (Leissner, 1972).

Another study concluded that

> there was no doubt that individual and social handicaps marched together remarkably closely . . . It does not follow, of course, that because they are found together that personal maladjustment is caused by poverty; on the contrary, it could be argued that, under present day conditions, to be conspicuously poorer than one's neighbour is a consquence of personal inadequacy (West, 1969).

While favourable socio-economic conditions do not necessarily ensure that children's psychological needs are met, it is much more difficult to do so in circumstances of severe socio-economic strain.

Moreover, to be able to give and receive love it needs to have been experienced and many parents have themselves been unloved if not rejected in childhood.

The need for security may also remain unsatisfied because parental behaviour is unpredictable and contradictory. On the one hand, discipline tends to be autocratic; also physical punishment may at times be more of an outlet for parental anger and frustration, generated by the pressures of the daily struggle rather than a means of ensuring the child's conformity to desired standards of behaviour. Chastisement of this kind only succeeds in teaching its recipient to respect and to use force himself; even a verbal berating, coupled with threats of being 'put away', is more likely to make a child feel rejected than to enable him to understand what is expected of him and why.

On the other hand, living in a state of perpetual crisis and chronic frustration, the parents' capacity to deal with their own anxieties is often so limited that they feel helpless and overwhelmed by the problems of sheer existence. Hence they are unable to provide the necessary emotional support to their children at times of anxiety and conflict. Yet the children are in great need of such support just because family stability is inevitably so precarious.

The pressures of life in the most disadvantaged homes also prevent the parents from being adequate models for their children. The unskilled labourer, whose earnings are low and irregular and who leaves all family responsibilities to his wife; the mother who scorns or fears him, and who is herself weighed down by the burden of home-making and child-rearing – neither is able to present a picture of adult life and behaviour which is likely to evoke their children's respect or a desire to become like them. Worse still, as the children grow into adolescence they will become increasingly aware of how limited their chances are of escaping from the constricting net of their multiple disadvantages.

Thus many youngsters from severely disadvantaged families, being thrown back upon their own resources, come to look to their siblings and to their peers in the street for emotional support and for model figures. Is it justified to argue that turning to contemporaries and to gang life because parental support is so limited, shows early independence and self-sufficiency? At the same time, when faced with outside criticism, such youngsters show highly ambivalent attitudes, expressing strong feelings of family loyalty and affection. Probably this is because they have never known security or acceptance elsewhere. It is similar to the loyalty shown by children who have been neglected or even abused by their parents. 'The attachment of children to parents who by all ordinary standards are very bad is a never-ceasing source of wonder to those who seek to help them' (Bowlby, 1951).

Having had to adapt to precarious relationships as well as inconsistent or otherwise unsatisfactory parental models, and having lacked a predictable framework of discipline, the child will expect other authority figures, such as teachers, to behave in a similar fashion.

Because his needs for new experience, and for praise and recognition will probably have been inadequately met too, he comes to school ill-prepared to respond to what will be demanded of him. Even if aware of the value of play and of fostering language development, his parents will rarely have had the emotional or physical resources to provide either to a satisfactory degree. A limited range of experiences and limited language skills will make him an unrewarding, because unresponsive, pupil. From the outset, he confronts his teachers with both behaviour and educational difficulties so that they may soon come to expect low standards from him while he will be aware of their disappointment in him. And so all too often their mutual expectations will eventually become self-fulfilling prophecies.

He in turn will be bewildered by the, to him, alien achievement-orientated climate of the class-room; by the conflicting standards of behaviour expected at home and at school; by the displeasure and disappointment shown by his teacher towards his ineffective efforts; and by her disapproval and punishment of his lack of progress. Her assessment of him as 'hopeless' will make him feel 'hopeless' too. And so he may well come to view school life with the same attitude of resigned or resentful helplessness with which his parents view their own fate. Thus his educational experience only confirms the attitudes formed earlier by parental handling:

> unable to identify with or to beat the system, he will expect nothing nor will he be equipped to do anything about it. Thus the child born into the lowest social bracket has everything stacked against him, including his parents' principles of child upbringing (Newson, 1972).

The fourth need, for responsibility, is often forced upon the child prematurely. He may have to fend for himself, both before going to school and when returning to an empty house afterwards. If there is a large family, he may have to assume pseudo-parental roles by taking care of younger siblings, to the detriment of his own development. When he fails to control them or when accidents occur he is likely to incur punishment. Yet he is given little chance to exercise responsibility appropriate to his age and ability level and with appropriate adult guidance.

Thus, on the one hand, being given responsibility is likely to be a source of anxiety and a burden, instead of an enjoyable opportunity which becomes increasingly challenging with age. On the other hand, in terms of his own personal life, his freedom of choice will be severely circumscribed by his lack of educational skills and social know-how. At best, a boring, poorly paid job with few prospects and fewer opportunities for exercising responsibilities lies ahead. At worst, there will be unemployment with its destructive effect on self-respect and self-confidence.

Social handicap and delinquency

Though the total and abject poverty of fifty years ago is now rare, today's greater general affluence may make a barren life and relative deprivation more difficult to bear: when the ownership of material possessions is widely advertised and equated with the good life; when having fun at parties, on yachts and at exotic beaches abroad, is featured prominently as the desirable way to spend one's leisure; then is it not likely that the dull, dead streets of inner cities and of redevelopment areas, as well as the windy deserts below high-rise tower blocks, feel even duller, deader and more frustrating by comparison? When everyone is poor or in danger, a shared fate makes for fellow feeling and solidarity. The more glaring the inequalities, the greater the divisiveness, resentment and hostility.

Yet, contrary to public fears, the majority of youngsters from severely disadvantaged homes are not angry and militant but apathetic and unassertive.

> Far from challenging the world around them, they seem personally and socially incarcerated; their talents are consistently under-rated, their vision constricted, their most personal modes of expression stifled. Each self-image they have created for themselves has been repeatedly deflated, all futures prematurely and permanently foreclosed (Davies, 1969).

On the other hand,

For statistical purposes, basic social factors will undoubtedly prove the most effective predictors of delinquency, but cause and effect is another matter. This Study has also shown the remarkable concentration of parental pathology, in the shape of unsuitable discipline, unfortunate attitudes to children, personality deviations, etc., among the socially handicapped group. Personal inadequacies and external handicaps reinforce each other in these unfortunate families. Rather than trying to answer the conundrum 'Which comes first . . .?' it may be more useful to ask at what point to try to break the vicious circle (West, 1969).

HANDICAPPED CHILDREN

How well a handicapped child makes out in the long run depends far less on the nature, severity or onset of his condition than on the attitudes of his parents first and foremost, then on those of his peers and teachers, and eventually on society's. These determine how he feels about himself and his handicap. This has been confirmed by many studies (Pringle and Fiddes, 1970; Dinnage, 1971 and 1972; Pilling, 1972 and 1973; Younghusband et al., 1970; Pringle, 1965 and 1970; Walker, 1982). It is illustrated too by the vivid biographies of those who have triumphed over severe disabilities (such as Carlson, 1952; Brown, 1954; Eareckson, 1978; Hill, 1976; Hickford, 1977; Kaufman, 1976; Munday, 1976).

Difficulties in meeting basic psychological needs

In essence the needs of the handicapped are the same as those of normal children but the presence of a disability poses some special problems. These will first be considered in relation to the basic psychological needs outlined earlier (see Chapter 2).

Love and security To give a sense of security one needs to feel secure oneself. But this is just what many parents of a handicapped child do not feel: most are worried by their lack of special knowledge and afraid of being unable to meet his special needs; many feel guilty or ashamed: some may be completely at a loss, especially those parents of slow learning children who themselves are of limited ability and weighed down by all the demands of modern life. Inevitably there is less support from and sharing with relatives and friends since they also lack the experience of bringing up a handicapped child.

At school, too, special difficulties are likely to arise in meeting this need unless the child is among the lucky few for whom an early and correct diagnosis is made, a place is available in a suitable school (whether ordinary or special) and long-term educational guidance, in the fullest sense of the term, is provided throughout his school life.

If his disability is not recognised and he tries to hold his own with normal children, he will come to feel inferior and a failure, the more so the less obvious or easily understood the nature of his handicap. To the blind and to some kinds of physical handicap, sympathy is readily extended; mental handicap is more often met with ridicule or contempt. If his teacher lacks knowledge of and experience with handicapped children, she may feel unable to cope adequately; if in addition she is faced with a large class, it is not surprising that a handicapped pupil may seem to her, and thus feel himself to be, a severe burden.

That parents feel concerned, and often extremely anxious, about their handicapped child is entirely natural. This concern could be harnessed to provide the motivation for giving that extra care, time and thought to the handicapped child which can help him to overcome, as far as possible, the adverse effects of his disability. Instead, this concern often turns into over-anxiety or resentment: if left without any clear idea about the nature of the disability and its short- as well as long-term implications, parental uncertainty may show itself in insecure and inconsistent handling of the child. The more severe, complex or multiple the handicap, the more urgent it is to provide continuous supporting services for parents.

Adequate facilities for a comprehensive initial diagnosis and for periodic re-assessments would also greatly contribute to meeting the handicapped child's need for security. When parents and teachers understand his particular condition, they convey this to him by their confident and continuous encouragement and support. A happy, harmonious community – be it the family or a school staff – communicates warmth, confidence and hope to the child instead of anxiety, uncertainty or hopelessness (Pugh and Russell, 1977).

The need for new experiences Here the handicapped child is inevitably at a disadvantage since a disability delays or even makes impossible the acquisition of some new experiences. As yet little is known about how different disabilities distort learning. For example, the physically handicapped may fail to acquire adequate experience of space and movement which will affect concepts of distance, of dimension and later of mathematics. The deaf all too often remain unstimulated by speech and language until much later than normal children, and even then benefit to a more limited extent; hence they may fail to acquire an adequate basis for abstract thought. Slow learning children are unable to benefit from new experiences at the time that normal children do; thus they may miss the opportunity for learning altogether if these experiences are not deliberately provided at a later stage than is usual; and the blind can never know the physical attributes of the world around them in the way the sighted majority do.

Not only is a distortion of learning difficult to prevent, it is also inevitably cumulative and progressive. The precise ways in which it affects the quality of learning have so far been little explored. Meanwhile the ingenuity of parents and teachers will be taxed to the full by trying to provide and adapt new experiences to the child's limitations without curtailing the range of these experiences more than is absolutely necessary.

Modifications may be required in the order and manner in which new experiences are presented; more careful grading and specially devised tools and apparatus may have to be used to ensure progress. Otherwise, new experiences may become a source of anxiety and defeat instead of an exciting challenge (Wall, 1979).

One effective way of learning, open to all handicapped children, except the deaf, is through speech. For some, such as the blind and physically severely disabled, it is a compensatory way of broadening their experience and understanding. Hence talking to and encouraging the child to speak from the earliest age are particularly important.

The need for recognition and achievement Here the handicapped face twin difficulties because of two tacit assumptions. First, praise habitually given for achievement rather than effort. This is at best unjust and positively harmful at worst. For example, writing a few lines of composition will cost a physically handicapped child a great deal more in terms of concentration and effort than it does the normal child to produce twice as much; yet the latter is more likely to be commended for his work. Secondly, the success of the handicapped tends to be judged by the extent to which their achievements approximate to those of the normal majority. In consequence, the more severe the handicap, the less likely is it that the child will be rewarded, genuinely and unreservedly, by recognition and a sense of achievement.

Thus to meet this need, we must grant the handicapped the fulfilment of another, specific to them, 'the need to be different and the need to be the same' (Mallinson, 1956). This means recognising that while they share the basic needs of all children, due allowance must be made for the differences imposed by the nature of a particular disability.

The need for responsibility The nature of a handicap may set a limit to the ultimate degree of responsibility a child will become capable of exercising. However, too low a limit may be set from a sense of pity or over-protection, or else through underestimating what he might become able to achieve, given the opportunity and necessary support. Also, one must guard against a whole household revolving around the handicapped child; rather he should be given the opportunity, both at home and in school, to shoulder some responsibilities, however limited in scope, so that he learns to give as well as to receive. In this way, self-respect and self-acceptance are fostered.

Social, emotional and educational adjustment

In recent years there has apparently been an increase in the number of children with multiple handicaps. To some extent this may stem, paradoxically enough, from the growth of medical knowledge: many babies are now surviving who would formerly have died (for example, those with spina bifida); and some conditions (such as retrolental fibroplasia or thalidomide limb deficiencies) were directly attributable to new treatment techniques. It may also be that an increasing understanding of, and attention to, potentially handicapping conditions as well as of their emotional and social concomitants is leading to their more effective recognition. In contrast, the development of appropriate treatment, educational and supportive facilities has lagged behind so that the complex needs of such children and their families are all too often inadequately met.

Since most disabilities burden the child with the additional handicap of distress or resentment about his condition, it is difficult to ascertain whether and to what extent any difficulties in behaviour, learning or adaptation are primarily 'organic' in origin. However, a few generalisations are justified on the basis of the literature reviews, covering the past fifteen years, which have been carried out by the Bureau (Pringle, 1967 and 1969; Dinnage, 1971 and 1972; Dinnage, 1986a, b, c, d and e; Dinnage and Gooch, 1986f).

What are the effects of different handicaps on adjustment and attainment? Blindness alone does not seem to be an insurmountable obstacle to the achievement of emotional or intellectual maturity. Blind children are able to reach the same standards as the sighted although they have to make prolonged and intense effort to develop abilities which come easily to the sighted. There is no research evidence that they are aided in this by any special compensatory faculties or attitudes. Parental support and understanding, as well as good intellectual ability in the child, appear to be the most crucial factors. Additional mental and physical handicaps – which are becoming more common in the blind child population – inevitably have detrimental consequences. Partially sighted children appear to be rather less well-adjusted than the blind and a higher proportion have educational difficulties.

Deafness, particularly if profound, almost always seriously impedes learning to communicate and to understand abstract thought; hence it restricts both intellectual and educational progress. More than any other handicap, except perhaps autism, it presents enormous barriers to the development of spontaneity and confidence in the parents towards the baby; and the child has to face similar barriers in building reciprocal relationships.

It is probable that the deep compassion aroused by blindness helps, just as the self-consciousness and irritation engendered by deafness hinder, good social, emotional and educational adjustments. Studies of those affected by orthopaedic handicaps and by thalidomide also highlight the central role of parental and society's attitudes. These determine how children cope with their difficulties far more than the severity of the actual deformity.

For example, of two seven-year-old thalidomide victims, one, a boy, was born without a left hand and the other, a girl, without arms and additionally unable to walk. Yet the girl was making good educational progress in an ordinary school where she had happy relationships with other children and with her teachers. The far less seriously handicapped boy showed signs of emotional disturbance and educational underfunctioning; however, his parents were over-protective while at the same time denying the existence of his deformity. The girl, on the other hand, was treated with loving care and compassionate but realistic common sense (Pringle and Fiddes, 1970).

This study also showed that though there has been much more emphasis on the limb deficiencies resulting from thalidomide, in fact many children suffered auditory impairment too; this had a much worse effect on intellectual ability, and on language and social development.

Among the cerebrally palsied the incidence of emotional, social and sensory difficulties is high. These are linked with intellectual and educational retardation as well as with a disturbed home background. After leaving school, only a minority, even of those whose physical disability is mild, lead normal social lives (Dinnage, 1986c).

There is a growing number of studies of the emotional, social, and educational adjustment of children with spina bifida, as many more of them have been able to survive owing to modern surgical and medical techniques. Results show that there is generally a constellation of difficulties dogging these children as they grow up (Dinnage, 1986b).

In summary, most comparative studies show the handicapped child to be less mature and more disturbed than those without disabilities; nevertheless, there is no evidence that maladjustment or educational retardation are inevitable. Where the nature of the handicap imposes severe limitations, whether physical or social, then behaviour and learning are bound to be affected. However, available data do not show any definite association between a particular disability and a particular behaviour characteristic. So much then for negative conclusions.

On the positive side, there seems to be general agreement that parental attitudes towards the child and his handicap are of paramount importance. A conclusion reached by some early American workers has remained undisputed to this day: 'The child seems to adopt the same attitude to the disability that his parents do. If they worry about it, so does he. If they are ashamed of it, he will be sensitive too. If they regard it in an objective manner, he will accept it as a fact and will not allow it to interfere with his adjustment' (Allen and Pearson, 1928). This view has been endorsed by Carlson (1952), who himself succeeded in triumphing over severe physical disability; moreover, by becoming a doctoi, he achieved a breakthrough in the attitudes to, and the treatment of, his own disability, cerebral palsy: 'Success or failure does not depend on what we lack but rather upon the use we make of what we have'.

CHILDREN IN ONE-PARENT FAMILIES

So far there has been relatively little research into the psychological and social effects on children of growing up in one-parent families. These will naturally vary, not only because of individual differences between children, but also because the age when one parent has to take over and the period during which only one cared for the child are bound to have a differential effect. Some of these questions will be examined in the Bureau's ongoing study of one-parent families; and they have already been explored in relation to illegitimately born children in the national cohort.

There is much evidence that a considerable proportion of one-parent families are likely to suffer financial hardship, if not actual poverty (Holman, 1970; Marsden, 1969; Pochin, 1969; Wynn, 1964 and 1970). Less is known about the emotional, social and educational effects. Results obtained from the Bureau's *National Child Development Study* made it possible to show that economic circumstances vary not only in relation to which parent is bringing up the family but also with regard to the reason why this is so. The rates of payment made by the Supplementary Benefits Commission were chosen as the general indicator of a subsistence standard of living (Essen, 1978 and 1979; Ferri, 1976; Ferri and Robinson, 1976).

As many as one in nine children (or 11 per cent) were no longer being cared for by both their natural parents by the time they were eleven years old, according to the results of the Study. Of these, some 5 per cent were being raised by one parent alone; the other 6 per cent were being brought up in more than thirty different types of 'anomalous' family circumstances. Here three particular groups will be considered: those being brought up single-handed by one natural parent; those born illegitimate; and children of divorce.

Single-parent families

The children in the study who – for whatever reason – were living in a one-parent family at the age of eleven years were more likely to have lost their father than their mother. In fact, the proportion of fatherless children was nearly five times as high as those who grew up without a mother. Although the rate of re-marriage was very similar for fathers and mothers respectively (about a third in each case), a further 25 per cent of the motherless children were being cared for by a mother substitute whereas father substitutes were provided for only 5 per cent of the fatherless children (Ferri, 1976; Ferri and Robinson, 1976).

Thus women are much more likely than men to be left caring single-handed for their families, following the loss of their marriage partner. This probably reflects differences in social attitudes: much greater sympathy is extended to the man who has been deserted by his wife and is trying to look after the children; also grandmothers, sisters or neighbours are more ready to offer help. However, there is perhaps less acceptance of a father staying at home and living on state support. The deserted wife calls out far less concern and assistance. There is a tacit assumption that it is easier and perhaps also more appropriate for a woman to combine the parental and wage-earning role than it is for a man on his own to do so.

The most common single cause resulting in one natural parent being left to bring up a family was marital breakdown; in fact, divorce, separation and desertion accounted for about half the cases. In the remaining families, where there was no mother, this was due to her having died; in households without a father, death was the reason in only a third of cases; the rest consisted mainly of illegitimately born children whose mothers were raising them.

In 1969, when the children were eleven years old, almost half (47 per cent) of the fatherless families had been dependent on state support at some time during the preceding twelve months; this compares with only 6 per cent among intact families. Motherless children were less badly off although their families were twice as likely to have received Supplementary Benefits than two-parent homes. Even single-handed mothers who did not have to rely on state support were probably worse off financially than their male counterparts since women workers are usually paid at a much lower rate. Mothers whose husbands had died were far less likely to have had to rely on benefits than when the marriage had broken down or the child was illegitimate. These trends were still valid when the children were followed up at 16 years (Fogelman, 1983).

Examining the quality of housing in terms of the availability of basic amenities, twice as many fatherless as two-parent families lacked the sole use of a bathroom, indoor lavatory and hot water supply; the situation of motherless children was also less favourable but not quite as bad as that of the fatherless (Ferri, 1976).

Children born illegitimate

A marked increase in the proportion of illegitimate births has taken place during recent years; also more unmarried mothers are choosing to keep their babies. Yet until recently little was known about how the mothers and their children were faring, in the short or medium term; or whether illegitimacy continues to present personal and social problems, even though attitudes towards extra-marital sexual relations have changed.

The *National Child Development Study* made it possible to seek some answers to these questions by comparing an unselected national group of illegitimate children, born in 1958, with their peers born in the same week (Crellin, Pringle and West, 1971; Lambert and Streather, 1980). The findings clearly showed that to be born illegitimate is to be born 'at risk'.

As in other recent studies, there was no difference in social class background between mothers who have a legitimate and an illegitimate baby. However, the latter were at a potential disadvantage, right from the start, in respect of their mother's age and their own family position. There were five times as many very young mothers among the illegitimate and nearly twice as many were having their first child. Among both these groups, the perinatal mortality rate is higher as is the prevalence of low birth weight. The overall mortality rate and the proportion of low birth weight babies were in fact markedly higher among the illegitimately born.

Ante-natal care was also markedly poorer among mothers-to-be of the illegitimate. A higher proportion than among the legitimate did not seek such care or did so later than is advisable; and a higher proportion failed to make an advance booking for their delivery.

About a third of the illegitimately born babies were given up by their mothers for adoption; they were then being brought up in a much more favourable home environment than those who had remained with their own mothers. The development of these two groups, who had had a similar start in life, was compared when they were seven years old.

By that time, the majority of the illegitimately born was living in some kind of two-parent situation (including those who were adopted). However, a considerable number of homes lacked a stable father figure. Only one in four children lived with both their natural parents.

The most outstanding feature was the much more favourable situation of the adopted. Among the illegitimate not adopted many had to share household amenities or lacked them completely: in fact, this was twice as prevalent as among the whole legitimate group. The same was true of over-crowding, despite the fact that there was a high proportion of only children among the illegitimate.

A considerable number of children experienced supplementary or total substitute care. This was made necessary by the high proportion of mothers who worked outside the home before the child went to school, and by their difficult and unsettled family circumstances. Over three times as many illegitimate as legitimate children were placed in day care facilities; and this proportion is certain to be an underestimate. In the first place, nearly two-thirds of the mothers of illegitimate children worked before the latter went to school; yet only a quarter of the children were reported to have had day care. Even allowing for relatives helping out, a sizable discrepancy remains. Another reason is that information was lacking about child minders, whether officially registered or those with whom mothers had made some private arrangement.

The proportion of children who came into the care of a local authority or voluntary body was five times higher among the illegitimate than legitimate children.

It is evident, then, that the dice are still heavily loaded against the illegitimately born child. What were the effects on his development? In all aspects which were examined, consistent and marked differences were found between the illegitimate, the adopted and the legitimate group. Time and time again, the illegitimate were at the bottom of the league table, whether for general knowledge, oral ability, creativity, perceptual development, reading attainment or arithmetical skills.

Even in the relatively more favourable environment of middle-class homes, the illegitimate did less well than legitimate children in such homes. Over and above social class effects, there were important 'illegitimacy effects'. For example, they account for twelve months' difference in progress between the adopted and the illegitimate groups in reading. In contrast, the progress made by the adopted was similar to that made by legitimate children in the same social class.

Once they went to school the illegitimate also suffered disadvantages. They had more changes of school; their attendance was more irregular; and their parents showed less interest in their educational progress. Marked differences were also found between the three groups of children in behaviour and adjustment in school. The proportion of 'maladjusted' children was nearly twice as high among the illegitimate as the legitimate, while the adopted more closely resembled the latter.

Inevitably, many questions remain unanswered. For example, there was no information on the personality of the child's mother or other members of his family. Soon, however, it will be possible to say whether the problems encountered by the illegitimate differ from those who, for other reasons, live in one-parent families. Meanwhile, it is evident that illegitimacy still brings with it personal and social problems. The children were beset by a multiplicity of unfavourable circumstances; these gave them a relatively poorer start in life which continued to build up into a complex web of cumulative and interacting hardships and deprivations. To be born illegitimate is still to be born disadvantaged, at least for the present.

Can a favourable environment halt or reverse the effects of early disadvantage? To judge from the development of those children who were adopted, the answer is that it can. Of course, it remains to be seen what the later development will be of both those who were and those who were not adopted.

Children of divorce

Every year the family life of thousands of children is disrupted by divorce and since the 1960s the number has risen sharply. In 1968, the total number of children under sixteen who were affected by divorce was some 60,000; in 1971, largely due to the Divorce Reform Act of 1969, there was a 55 per cent increase in petitions and the number of children involved rose to 117,000, three-quarters of whom were under sixteen. By 1980, the number of children under sixteen whose parents divorced rose to a peak of 163,000 (Central Statistical Office, 1986). At present, it seems likely that one in five children will be affected before their sixteenth birthday (Office of Population Censuses and Surveys, 1983).

There may well be a link between the rising divorce rate and the increasing trend towards early parenthood which allows young couples little time to adjust to the new relationships and responsibilities of marriage; then financial and housing problems are added with the arrival of a baby. If both spouses are under twenty when they marry the divorce rate (in England and Wales) is about three times the rate for all marriages. 'One of the most striking demographic features associated with divorce is the increased risk among wives who were pregnant at the time of marriage . . . marriages are now taking place at a younger age than previously and young brides are forming an increasing proportion of all pre-marital pregnancies so it is likely that a larger number of children than at present will be innocent witnesses of a broken home and family' (Gibson, 1973).

Remarkably little attention has been given to the effects which the break-up may have on children's development. What research there is has largely been confined to self-selected and probably atypical groups, namely those seen in psychiatric and child guidance clinics. 'We do not know whether it damages the child least to grow up in an unhappy home with both parents, or alone with one parent where there is no remarriage, or with one parent and a step-parent' (Mortlock, 1972). In relation to children's reactions to new marriages of either of their parents it has been suggested that 'overall, it seems it is better to have three or even four parents and six grandparents than no father or mother. This pattern of multiple marriages in fact produces a new type of extended family and consequently a variety of people with whom the child can identify and form relationships' (Benn, 1969). But step-parenting can itself bring problems (Ferri, 1984).

Financially, there is often a drop in the standard of living since most children will stay with their mother who now depends on alimony which is not only a reduced but may also not be a reliable source of income. Even if she herself is earning a salary, it will be less than the previous joint income; moreover, she may have to incur additional expense in having the children looked after out of school hours and term time.

On the psychological side, it is difficult to help a child to understand the reasons for the marriage break-up, the more so the younger the child, and the more bitter the feelings between the parents. Not uncommonly they vie for the child's affections, blackening each other's character and motives in the process. At worst, the child may become a pawn in their game of mutual hurt and ascendancy which is played out during prolonged battles for custody; an extreme example being 'tug-of-love' children who are whisked from one home, and sometimes one country, to another in the fight for possession. (An even worse situation is a new phenomenon reported from the United States, namely that neither parent is willing to take on custody; such a degree of rejection is bound to have a most damaging effect on a child's sense of personal worth.) Even at best, when regular and frequent 'access' has been agreed so that the child spends some time with the parent who does not have custody, meetings at weekends and during holidays are not readily conducive to maintaining a close relationship.

What evidence there is suggests that a sizable proportion of children whose parents have been divorced show disturbed behaviour. Whether this is due as much, or more, to deteriorating relationships and possibly open quarrels prior to the final break-up of the marriage, or to the child's conflict of loyalties, or to the finality of the divorce itself, has not yet been established. What is agreed by many, including some lawyers, is that custody decisions, in the lower courts at any rate, tend to be arrived at too hastily and with too little attempt to take into account the child's own wishes or needs. If his long-term interests are to be regarded as of major importance, then some reform of divorce proceedings would seem essential.

CHILDREN LIVING APART FROM THEIR FAMILIES

The reasons why children have to live apart from their families range from parental inadequacy and intractable pathology to inability to cope with overwhelming circumstances; and from temporary crisis to permanent abandonment.

During the past twenty-five years, three major advances have been made in our understanding of the implications of substitute care for children. They are well supported by research, but none has yet been translated into action on the required scale. The first is that adequate physical care is not sufficient to ensure satisfactory emotional, social and intellectual growth; secondly, that prolonged institutional life in a children's home and especially in hospital can have very damaging effects on a child's all-round development; and thirdly that many, if not a majority, of children could remain in their own homes if effective and sufficient supportive services within the community were available.

To bring this about requires different social priorities and policies regarding housing, a minimum income and allowances for single parents as well as for handicapped children or adults. A discussion of these changes is outside our brief, but two official statistics clearly illustrate this fact: first, each year about half of all the children who come into care do so because of their mother's confinement or short-term illness. Secondly, chronic mental or physical illness, and desertion or death of one parent, account for a further 10 per cent of children. Research is needed to clarify how many children could be kept in their own homes, and how successfully, both in the short- and the long-term; and how best to plan for those who are in care (Parker, 1980).

A wide diversity of circumstances leads to the separation of children from their families. Are there, nevertheless, differences between them and other children of the same age and similar social background, who did not experience removal from homes; and what is the evidence that the former are more vulnerable? These questions will be examined in relation to three groups: those who have spent at least one period in residential care; or in foster care; or who have lived for long periods in hospital.

Children in residential care

The evidence quoted is based on four sources: first, reviews of literature in the United States, Western Europe, Israel and Great Britain covering the period from 1948 to 1974, carried out by the Bureau (Dinnage and Pringle, 1967; Prosser, 1976); second, a series of linked studies of seven-, eleven- and fifteen-year-olds (Pringle, 1971); thirdly, the Bureau's *NCDS* (Mapstone, 1969 and 1973; Essen, Lambert and Head, 1976); and lastly, a study of children needing substitute parents (Rowe and Lambert, 1973).

Social, family and personal background Are there any features which distinguish those children who, by the age of seven, have spent at least one period in care, from all the others in the *National Child Development Study*? It proved possible, in fact, to draw quite a distinctive picture of them even though there will, of course, be much individual variation within the 'in care' group.

To begin with, nine out of every ten came from working-class homes. This is not really unexpected. Though separation experiences and unsatisfactory mothering are not confined to any one social group, nevertheless middle-class parents, who are unable or unwilling to look after their children, can usually make their own arrangements for substitute care. Their solutions – a nanny, *au pair* girl or boarding school – are quite unlikely options for the manual worker.

Next, the 'in care' group tended to live in homes which were more crowded and had fewer amenities than those of children in the comparable social class who had not been in care. Also, they had more brothers and sisters, and this was the case irrespective of social class. They had, too, experienced more home moves and changes of school.

Perhaps even more significant, their disadvantages dated back to the time of their birth. Already, as they lay in their cots, the group of children who later were received into care could be distinguished from the other children born during the same week. More of them were born to unsupported mothers who were likely to be younger and of smaller stature; as babies, children tended to have had a shorter period of gestation and to be of lower birth weight. These characteristics are not, of course, independent of each other but, taken together, they indicate a group of children who were in these first few days of life already at a disadvantage compared with other children of the same age and social class.

Lastly, at seven years, proportionately more children who had been in care were short in height and light in weight for their age. In comparison with their classmates they appeared to their teachers to have poor control of their hands when writing, drawing or buttoning up their coats; they were fidgety; they tended to have poor physical coordination when running about, jumping, or throwing balls; they were clumsy; and hardly ever still. Their teachers also thought their appearance to be less attractive than that of the other children, one in five being said to look scruffy or very dirty, and one in ten underfed.

This group was not composed of long-stay, institutionalised children. Indeed about 25 per cent had had only one period in care, lasting four weeks or less; 66 per cent had been in care for no more than a year, even when there were several occasions. For most, the experience of being in care was of brief duration in relation to their total life span.

Thus the *National Child Development Study* results confirm that even children who come into short-term care, ostensibly because of their mother's confinement, tend to belong to socially disadvantaged families (Schaffer and Schaffer, 1968). Earlier findings have also shown that large families with low income, those where there is only one parent, or where there is physical or mental handicap, are at greater risk of disintegration, and that once a family is split up, reintegration may be difficult (Dinnage and Pringle, 1967). Hence, coming into care for the first time could be regarded as an early warning signal of a child's vulnerability.

Learning and behaviour difficulties Recovery from single, brief separation experiences has been shown to be fairly rapid. Therefore emphasis will here be given to the effects of long-term separations.

There is evidence of both language and intellectual retardation among infants and young children, which is the more serious the less adequate the psychological care (Dinnage and Pringle, 1967; Rutter, 1972). For example, a comparative study of four-year-olds showed both qualitative and quantitative differences: those in residential nurseries used smaller vocabularies, more immature sentence formations, expressed less fantasy and humour in their play or talk, and employed fewer active verbs. Also their knowledge of everyday domestic activities, such as cooking, was very limited and they were not even sure of the names of the various parts of their own bodies. The all-too-common absence of father figures, especially in homes for pre-school children, was reflected in their ignorance of male personal effects and apparel (Pringle, 1971).

Among children of school age, too, lower levels of language, intellectual and educational performance have been found in investigations carried out in the UK and elsewhere. Despite the fact that different research methods and different institutional settings have been used, there is considerable agreement that many children in long-term residential care function less well than their peers (Dinnage and Pringle, 1967; Prosser, 1976).

This has also been demonstrated in a series of linked studies of seven-, eleven- and fifteen-year-olds (Pringle, 1971). At all three age levels, both intellectual and reading skills were found to be below average but the most serious backwardness was in language development. Admission into care at an early age (i.e., pre-school) and subsequent lack of contact with adults outside the residential home seemed to have a particularly detrimental effect on both achievement and adjustment. A higher proportion than among the ordinary child population showed behaviour difficulties, both at school and in the children's home, the commonest symptoms being anxiety, restlessness and aggression.

These findings, too, have been confirmed by the *National Child Development Study*. Once again, overall as well as within each social class grouping, the 'in care' group were doing less well in every aspect which was examined. In general knowledge, ability to express themselves in conversation, reading and arithmetic, the proportion performing poorly was twice or three times as high among them than among their peers. As one might predict, a proportionately large number were thought to need special educational help, either now or within the next two years.

Their behaviour at home (or if in care at the age of seven, in their substitute home) was characterised by frequent irritability, by a tendency to 'fly off the handle', by being miserable or tearful, by destructiveness with their own and other people's belongings, by aggressiveness towards other children and by an inability to settle to anything for more than a few moments.

In school they showed similar behaviour difficulties. The most marked difference between those who had been, or were still, in care and the other children was in the proportion showing hostility, both to other children and to adults, and 'inconsequential behaviour', i.e., lacking concentration and persistence; the teachers also described them as being untidy, slapdash and careless over appearance and with belongings, and impervious to correction. Thus, a picture emerges of children who, compared with their peers, are unhappy, insecure and immature.

Personal identity and relationships However adverse a home, the child lives in familiar surroundings and is looked after, however inadequately, by familiar people. Being taken from it means the collapse of the world he has accepted and trusted as the only one he knows. The younger the child, the greater the distress at being removed to an unfamiliar environment. The more limited his understanding of verbal explanations, the greater is his likely bewilderment and the more difficult the task of restoring his sense of security; also he may feel it was his naughtiness which led to his being sent away.

The most damaging effect, however, is probably on the growth of self-awareness and the development of a sense of identity. 'He has no single person who shares his own most basic and important memories, no one to confirm whether these memories are in fact correct or figments of his imagination, no one to polish up a fading memory before it is too late. Such a deprivation seems so damaging that I am not at all sure that we can ever fully make up for it artificially' (Newson, 1971). Not only does the child in long-term care have no reliable past; equally devastating, he has no predictable future except that he will come out of care at the age of eighteen.

In the ordinary home, both the store of personal memories and the framework of a personal future are built up through frequent everyday references and continuing discussions of family affairs. 'When you were little you had fair hair' and 'when you are older you can help dad in the shop' are phrases which crop up regularly, their predictability being a source of strength because of their very familiarity. The sense of a personal past as well as of a future lend perspective and continuity which are the essence of acquiring a sense of identity.

The youngster who has spent the major part of his life in care is often uncertain about why he came into care, why changes in placement were made, why other children moved on and why staff left; he may not know the names of the various people who have looked after him, let alone their current whereabouts; the same is true regarding the children who shared his life for certain periods; nor does he know what the future is likely to hold since long-term plans are rarely made (Page and Clark, 1977). If he goes to boarding school, because of a physical or mental handicap, he may not even know until the end of each term in which children's home he will be spending his next holidays.

In consequence, children who have been deprived of a normal home experience difficulties, especially during adolescence and adulthood, in accounting for themselves. Ordinary personal questions such as 'where do your people live?' or 'what does your father do?' become loaded and embarrassing. In confused panic, inventions about imaginary relatives may be produced because the deprived youngster knows little or nothing about his own background. This adds to his feelings of insecurity in personal relations and may lead him either to shun them or to weave a web of lies when faced with the need to account for himself.

There is some evidence of the importance to the child of having at least one dependable and lasting relationship with an adult while in long-term institutional care (Pringle, 1971). Two groups of children were compared, one notably stable, the other severely maladjusted (according to four independently made assessments). All of them had been separated from their mothers before the age of five years and had spent the major part of their lives away from their own home; their ages ranged from five to fifteen years. The aim was to investigate possible reasons for the difference in their adjustment.

The most marked and consistent difference between them was in the amount of contact maintained with parents or parent substitutes: the stable children enjoyed a dependable, lasting relationship in contrast to the maladjusted group, where only one child had done so; also most of the latter had been separated from their mothers very early (within the first year of life), so that they had not had the opportunity of forming bonds prior to admission into care. Hence the maladjusted group had neither established nor maintained stable relationships and their outstanding characteristic was an inability to make relationships with adults or children. A second study confirmed these findings.

Three hypotheses could account for the findings. First, the maladjusted group might have been constitutionally inferior and hence more susceptible to emotional instability; however, there was little evidence to support this view. Secondly, their very early and virtually permanent separation might have done irreparable harm to their basic personality structure. This view of emotional development has been criticised as being too sweeping, narrow and deterministic (Clarke and Clarke, 1973; Rutter, 1972; and Wootton, 1959). At the same time, knowledge is lacking on whether there is in fact a point of no return if the child remains permanently deprived of a close personal relationship with an adult.

The third hypothesis holds that, although prolonged and early separation and residential life are disturbing and potentially damaging experiences, this is not inevitably so. The opportunity to maintain continuous, frequent and regular contact with an adult outside the institution appeared to enable many a child to cope with them. This was so even when his own family had been indifferent or rejecting, and when he had never lived permanently with the parental substitute (i.e., only for weekends and holidays). What seemed crucial was that someone cared sufficiently to maintain a stable, enduring relationship.

It looks then as if – at least in our type of society – a child needs to feel that he matters as an individual; that he is valued for his own sake and not only by someone who is paid for the job of caring for him fairly and impartially. If lasting and unconditional love and loyalty from an adult are never experienced, then the child may fail to develop these qualities; also the later he learns to establish such relationships, the more difficult and longer it will be before he learns to trust adults and eventually reciprocate affection. Thus a vicious circle is likely to develop; not having known a secure relationship, the child fails to learn in early infancy the responses appropriate and expected in such a relationship.

The effects of institutional life

Clearly children who come into care, even for a short period only, are not a random group. Prior to separation, the majority live in homes where verbal stimulation is minimal: over-worked and under-privileged mothers, often burdened with too many pregnancies or forced by economic necessity to go out to work, have little time and energy available to encourage the baby in his early experiments with sound and to elicit continued trial and effort by taking delight in his pre-speech vocalisations; similarly, once the child is beginning to speak, there is likely to be less verbal stimulation in the form of nursery rhymes, stories, songs and general conversation.

When the child enters an institution, the staff-child ratio as well as the training of the staff are of paramount importance: too low a staffing ratio and an over-emphasis on child training as against child development, are all likely to have a retarding effect on the growth of language. Furthermore, less than 4 per cent of all residential staff are fully trained for their woık, and 62 per cent are totally untrained (Jones, 1973).

Being separated and having to live apart from their family for a time will then, at best, be another unsettling and, at worst, a deeply disturbing and damaging experience. Indeed, some may become the most disadvantaged group within each social class. It is difficult, if not impossible, to isolate and estimate separation effects from all the other unfavourable influences to which these children have been exposed. Also, the 'in care' experience itself will be different for each child, depending on his age, the length of time away from home, how often he was removed the quality of the substitute care provided, whether he remained in touch with members of his family or others close to him, as well as on his own resilience under stress.

On coming into care, establishing a bond of affection could help the child to regain self-confidence, but this requires time and continuity of daily handling. Many, if not most, residential nurseries and homes are unable to provide either. The rate of staff turnover also militates against their providing long-term relationships. The effects of this are well documented by now. Young children who remain in institutions tend to crave affection, to cling to visitors and later on to make indiscriminate friendships and to have difficulty in forming lasting relationships. Early and prolonged institutional care has also been shown to militate against successful fostering later on.

When in later life he is offered affection, he does not know how to reciprocate. His reactions will be immature, like those of a very young infant who naturally takes love for granted and demands unceasing devotion. In a normal family, the child learns as he grows older that he is expected to reciprocate: by delaying his demands for immediate or exclusive attention; by controlling his anger and selfishness; by considering the feelings of others; and by conforming to social expectations.

Not having learned all this at the usual time, the emotionally deprived child will later alienate and often lose any affection and goodwill offered because he seems selfish, greedy and ungrateful. This deprives him of the opportunity to learn the very skills needed in making close human relationships; instead he learns to mistrust affection when offered. Because of this mistrust, coupled with his emotional immaturity, he is likely to grow increasingly unable to respond when offered further opportunities for building up close, emotional ties. The more his ability to respond becomes stunted, the more his chances to build a reciprocal relationship recede. Eventually the vicious circle is closed: unloved and friendless, he is in turn unloving and hostile towards others.

Susceptibility to maladjustment and resilience in the face of rejection appear to depend on the quality of relationships available to the child while in care. By themselves, neither physical separation from the family nor living for long periods in institutions necessarily lead to emotional or learning difficulties.

Since most children coming into care are already disadvantaged socially, backward intellectually or educationally, and disturbed emotionally, it is insufficient for residential life to provide simply good physical care. If that is all, any positive gain is likely to be limited. Indeed, there is a danger that the 'cure', i.e., coming into care, will make the 'disease', i.e., being disadvantaged, even worse, because being in care itself has adverse effects. Only if children's institutions become 'therapeutic communities', aiming to remedy and rehabilitate the hurt, confused and damaged child, can they claim to provide a viable form of substitute care (Pringle, 1978a).

Children in limbo Are there children in the care of local authorities or voluntary agencies whose return to their families is uncertain or even unlikely? At a time when couples wanting to adopt greatly outnumber available children, one might have expected to find very few who need a permanent substitute family, living instead in long-term residential care. American work had shown that there are children who could have been placed in adoptive homes soon after they came into care; yet despite no real parental ties, they remained in institutions for so long that the likelihood of their being acceptable for adoption became remote. A pilot study in this country suggested that the same may be happening here (Laker and Tongue, 1972). Once again, the reason seems to be that greater weight is given to the (sometimes hypothetical) long-term interests of the parents rather than the child. Now the results of a more extensive study show that at least 17 per cent of children in long-term care need substitute parents (Rowe and Lambert, 1973).

The study covered thirty-three different voluntary or statutory agencies and examined nearly 3,000 children under the age of eleven years who had been in care for at least six months. In fact, over half of those aged between five and eleven years had already been in care for more than four years. Almost two thirds of the whole group were expected by their social worker to have to remain in care until they were eighteen years old; 80 per cent had been admitted under the age of five and 50 per cent before they were two years old. Half of all the children were illegitimate. Almost half had no contact at all with either parent, and for a further third it was infrequent (76 per cent altogether); less than one in four children saw one or both parents once a month or more often.

This then is the situation of children who are in need of substitute parents. Not unexpectedly, a very high proportion was reported to have behaviour problems and to be below average intelligence. One cannot help but wonder to what extent these difficulties are the consequence of long periods in care combined with minimal parental interest or contact.

The obstacle to placement most frequently mentioned by the social workers concerned was the presence of brothers or sisters; this would have meant finding a home willing to take more than one child. However, the study concludes that

> in most agencies the main problem in homefinding was pressure of other work. In many areas only crisis work could be done because of inadequate staff and resources in the face of rising demand for social services of all kinds. Stereotyped reviews and inadequate recording were often noted...and decisions about placement had often been delayed for long periods while efforts were made to solve the family's problems or while new staff became familiar with the case...only about one child in three had been under the supervision of the same social worker during the two years preceding the study and one in five had had more than three social workers during this time.

Translated into national terms, the authors estimate that there are probably about 7,000 children waiting to be placed in a foster or adoptive home. Yet there are grounds for suspecting that the study underestimates the real size of the problem: the information was based on the judgement of social workers who by training and experience tend to be adult-centred; this tendency appears to have been further increased by a number of recent trends, including the Seebohm reorganisation of social services and the politically fashionable emphasis on 'parental rights'. In consequence, there is a reluctance to assume such rights even on behalf of children whose parents have not been in touch with them for years and whose whereabouts cannot be traced. Yet available evidence strongly indicates that if a child has been in continuous care for a period of six months, he is very likely to remain there until he leaves school.

May it perhaps bring about a much-needed change in attitude if the concept of 'parental duties' was substituted? A parent who disappeared without subsequently making any effort to find out about his child's well-being or even whereabouts for, say, twelve or eighteen months would then automatically be considered to have abrogated his parental responsibilities rather than having to be sought by social agencies for months or years as is current practice. This would free a considerable number of children for long-term foster care or, better still, adoption.

Foster care

Much of what has been said about residential care applies also to those in foster care. Reviewing the literature, the most outstanding feature is the paucity of basic knowledge (Dinnage and Pringle, 1967; Prosser, 1978). There is no nationally agreed policy or comparability of practice. There are very wide variations from one part of the country to another in the proportion of children being fostered (from 22 to 60 per cent); and so, not surprisingly, it is still as true as it was ten years ago that fostering is 'an important but nevertheless unpredictable part of the resources available for caring for children' (Parker, 1966). Worse still, evidence regarding private fostering indicates that there is an inverse relationship between the unsuitability of foster parents and the amount of supervision given by social workers (Holman, 1973).

Many of the disadvantages and difficulties encountered by children in long-term residential care will apply to those who have been fostered since they, too, have lacked family support and stability; indeed, many of them have been in residential care as well. But while 'institutionalisation' has been defined and described, this is not so far 'fosterisation'. There is no profile of the typical foster child and such studies as there are, have largely been concerned with failure rather than success. Similarly, little is known about the 'good', i.e., unbroken, long-term, successful foster placement or even whether the unbroken placement is generally or even necessarily 'good'.

Why should this be so? The chief reason may be the very complexity of the process, both administratively and psychologically. There is much more uncertainty and impermanence than in adoption; and the involvement is closer, more personal and intimate than in residential care. Some of the complexity arises from the rather ill-defined roles of, and relationships between, all concerned:

the child who is being placed; his parents; the foster parents; and the placing agency's caseworker. Furthermore the assumptions, expectations and needs of each are widely different. So it is perhaps not unexpected that conflicting perceptions of the foster care situation have continued to exist for close to a hundred years and to this day there is no consensus (Cooper, 1978; D.H.S.S., 1981).

The following facts are supported by some evidence but all need substantiation: the first two years in foster care appear to be decisive in terms of both negative breakdown and positive rehabilitation; the younger the child when first fostered, the greater the likelihood that the placement will be a 'stable, successful' arrangement; the longer the child has been in institutional care during the first three years of life, the more likely fostering is to break down; this is the case, too, the older the child was when first separated from his mother; the breakdown rate is also related to the child's being emotionally disturbed, which in turn may well be due to his background and history, and in particular to rejection by parental figures.

As in so many other areas of development, sex differences are in the expected direction: boys have a higher incidence of behaviour difficulties and (possibly because of this) a higher rate of breakdown in their foster placements. Children of ethnic minorities are liable to have additional difficulties, relating to identification with white foster parents.

An understanding of the meaning of foster care, and of the reasons which made it necessary, seems to have a positive influence on the foster child's adjustment. This one would expect both from developmental and clinical studies of emotionally damaged children which suggest that harmful consequences are likely when a child is kept in ignorance (or told half-truths) about his origin or about his own family. Coming to terms with illegitimacy or with a parent's being in prison, mentally ill or having disappeared altogether is inevitably distressing; yet this knowledge is less harmful than living in a depersonalised vacuum, created by passive silence or by active concealment.

Much more needs to be known about the actual feelings of the children and adults involved in fostering. Qualitative studies of successful placements are especially lacking; as are studies of how 'vulnerable' groups, such as bereaved children, adolescents and school leavers make out in foster homes. The criteria determining placements, the processes involved in decision-making, and community attitudes to fostering also repay study. We need to assess, too, the experiments carried out by local authorities in recent years in using salaried foster-parents for certain types of placement. The danger of exploitation and wrong motivation undeniably exists, but inadequate remuneration is no guarantee against either; nor are affection and money mutually exclusive. Indeed, 'love alone is not enough' in caring for someone else's disturbed, if not damaged, child (Pringle, 1978).

Lastly, two kinds of longitudinal study are needed. First, a kind of 'natural history of foster parenthood': foster parents learn, and hence change, as they gain experience and understanding through their relationships with a variety of foster children, their parents and case workers. The nature of these changes will have implications for selection procedures and for the rate of successful placements. One such study is now available (Fanshel and Shinn, 1978).

Secondly, a longitudinal study, comparing foster children with those who have mainly been in residential care as well as with those who have lived with their own families would be valuable. One such project is part of the *NCDS* and some preliminary results are available (Mapstone, 1973). By the age of seven years, some 60 per cent of all the children who had been in care had experienced fostering. Of these, 53 per cent had been placed in two, and 8 per cent in three or more, different foster homes; 20 per cent had remained in the same foster home for one year or longer, and a further 25 per cent between two to eleven months; in the great majority of cases (86 per cent), the natural and foster parents did not meet nor did either of the natural parents visit the child while he was in foster care; over 40 per cent of mothers neither wrote to the child nor phoned the foster mother during the placement. These findings seem contrary to what is held to be good foster care practice.

The chronically handicapped child in hospital care

If it is difficult to satisfy a child's basic psychological needs while he lives in residential care, this is infinitely more difficult in long-stay hospitals. Their organisation, ethos, daily routine and staff training are in no way geared to do so. Acceptance of this fact has been very slow. Over twenty-five years ago it was advocated that long-stay hospitals should be reformed so that children lived in small groups under a housemother, and from there went to their lessons in a school, to their treatment in a sick-bay and to their entertainment in a central hall. There would be no disadvantage in the housemother having had a nursing training, but that in itself is not the qualification for the work she will do. Her duty is to live with her group of children and attempt to provide the things of which they have been deprived (Spence, 1947).

Some progress has, of course, been made. First, it has been recognised that thousands of children, who are chronically handicapped, mentally, physically or both, need not be in hospitals at all; this is necessary only because there are additional problems, connected with their home circumstances or with difficulties relating to special school placement. Several studies of mentally handicapped children have demonstrated this, but there are few comparable systematic accounts of physically handicapped children living in long-stay hospitals.

Secondly, some hospitals have over the years introduced more or less major reforms. Thirdly, a few experimental small units have been established, especially designed to replace hospital care altogether. Yet it is argued that 'what is needed is not wholesale closure of hospitals, but the recognition of their uniqueness and a reappraisal of their structure and function. Deprived and handicapped children need homes not wards. They need nursing in the widest sense, partly nursing, partly educational, and always parental' (Whalley, 1973).

A recent account of long-stay hospitals questions whether 'we have really advanced very much in the last hundred years when we tolerate the existence of forgotten, hidden children' (Oswin, 1971). The study highlights how inadequate an environment such hospitals are: the children are deprived of a mother-substitute, because care is fragmented and because staff changes are made deliberately (i.e., a three-monthly rota for nurses); they are deprived of play opportunities and of experiences outside the hospital walls; of a reasonable daily routine; of privacy and dignity when their physical needs are attended to; of pleasant meal-times which should be social occasions; and of achieving even a small degree of independence.

In short, the traditional way of treating the sick continues to be applied to the chronically handicapped.

Children cared for in a hospital ward regime tend to become depersonalised...the hierarchical medical and nursing approach is detrimental to their emotional, social and intellectual development...

those without a parent or guardian should be received into the care of the local authority while remaining in hospital, and all unvisited children should have a 'friend' appointed for them (Younghusband et al., 1970).

Weekend fostering for those whose parents cannot or will not have them home could provide at least some experience of ordinary family life.

There is then much evidence that even in good but large institutions the care provided differs both in quantity and quality from that in a family setting; and that the younger the child on admission and the longer he then remains institutionalised, the more likely that many aspects of his development will be adversely affected. Some experimental schemes have been introduced and monitored, showing that the ill-effects can be minimised or even avoided, provided major changes are made in institutional policy as well as in the daily regime (Tizard, 1972; Gibson, 1969). Also, the experience of the Kibbutz indicates that communal life in childhood does not inevitably lead to harmful consequences.

There is, however, no evidence for the view that 'better a bad family than a good institution'. Children's development is so gravely at risk in the worst families – which reject, ill-treat or batter the child – that even an institutional upbringing may be preferable. But this is anyhow a false antithesis since other alternatives are available for those requiring long-term or permanent substitute care.

BELONGING TO A MINORITY GROUP

In contrast to the various circumstances considered previously, belonging to a minority group is not in itself necessarily stressful. It will, however, become so when prejudice against a group is prevalent. A child belonging to it will become aware of the stigma or discrimination which may make his loyalty all the fiercer or may lower his self-esteem or possibly both. While little is known about the effects on emotional, social and intellectual development of feeling singled out in this way, it is likely to make a child more vulnerable, particularly if there are other stresses too.

Two very different conditions will be selected for discussion, namely being adopted and belonging to a racial minority. Though adoption still arouses some prejudice, it is not necessarily 'discovered' by outsiders, since it is an 'invisible' handicap. In contrast, looking racially different is in our society a most visible means of recognition from birth onwards. The social attitudes towards, and assumptions about, these two minority groups are complex and highly charged emotionally; also both exert their influence from a very early age through parental reactions to the stress of facing prejudice.

Adopted children

To begin with, the inability to have children is for many couples a source both of sorrow and reproach. If a sense of personal inadequacy persists in either partner, this will affect their attitude to each other and also, directly or indirectly, to the child. Next, many adoptive parents have to come to terms with their own, and later their adopted child's attitude to illegitimacy. Though disapproval of it may be lessening and though it is not always explicit or even conscious, this in no way detracts from its potency. As long as it exists in the community, neither the adopted child nor the adoptive parents can entirely escape its influence, even if they themselves do not share the prejudice.

Another difficulty relates to the concept of the 'blood tie'. Because considerable importance continues to be ascribed to it, both in popular and even legal thinking, adoption is seen very much as a second best. This is likely to be conveyed to the child. Similarly, the myth about morals being inherited is still believed by many; because many adopted children have been born illegitimate, adoptive parents tend to be fearful, especially during adolescence and in relation to girls, of immorality and promiscuity. Such fears about the effects of poor heredity can then become self-fulfilling prophecies. In fact, practically all studies have shown that the most important conditions for a successful adoption are the kind of home and care which the adopters are providing for the child.

Right from before birth, children who will later be adopted, are likely to be subjected to stressful influences. Many are conceived in an insecure environment and are carried by mothers who are beset by problems, so that their pregnancy will be a stressful period. This can have adverse effects even while the baby is still in utero. Then, both the mother who relinquishes her child and the prospective adopters have, for different reasons, to cope with many more doubts and anxieties than are faced by ordinary families (Seglow,

Pringle and Wedge, 1972, Chap. 17). Thus during the early months of life the baby may have been exposed to an anxiety-laden atmosphere. He may share not only the vulnerability of illegitimately born children but experience additional stress compared with those who remain with their own mothers. Also, he may have had several changes in mothering while awaiting adoption.

One further set of potentially stressful circumstances relates to the way in which the meaning of adoption is conveyed to the child, and what and how he is told about his biological parents. It is difficult to explain the necessary facts, while also maintaining as satisfactory an image as possible of the natural parents, and without implying that they rejected him. Equally difficult is 'the double bind of "make the child your own but tell him he isn't" . . . "telling" is inevitably seen as setting in motion complex and emotion-laden wheels which must change the family dynamics and which may create problems for the growing child' (Rowe, 1970). Awareness of these dilemmas can lead to a reluctance to discuss his origin, so that it becomes a topic shrouded in uneasy embarrassment or, worse still, unmentionable mystery. Such a situation is calculated to lead to intense curiosity, or even obsession, during adolescence.

In view of these potential difficulties, the high proportion of successful adoptions is all the more remarkable. Available research evidence shows that 'adoption is one of the soundest, most lasting – and incidentally cheapest – ways of meeting the needs of certain children who are socially deprived and in need of a normal home life' (Jacka, 1973). In fact, it is the most satisfactory form of permanent care yet devised by Western society for children whose own parents cannot undertake it (Witmer et al., 1963; Pringle, 1966, Kadushin, 1970; Seglow et al., 1972; Bohman and Sigvardsson, 1985). Its success also shows that loving care and a favourable environment can overcome, or even reverse, the effects of a whole range of early disadvantages and stresses (Tizard, 1977).

Children of ethnic minorities

The position of minority cultures in any society is often a difficult one. They can be confronted by racist attitudes and consequential adverse material and social circumstances. The children of ethnic minorities may in this sense be vulnerable in ways which can disadvantage their education, health or social welfare.

Studies reported earlier make clear the relationship between, for example, low family income and poor housing on the one hand, and children's poor attainment in school on the other. Whilst it can not be assumed that the same kind of relationship would necessarily hold for all ethnic groups, such adverse material circumstances are certainly ones which should alert us to the likelihood of increased vulnerability in their children. More subtle and pervasive are the effects of any lowered expectations of adults, particularly teachers, upon the child's performance or development.

The vulnerability of some children from minority cultures is often linked to the gap between the language or form of English used in the home or neighbourhood, and the language of the school. This is not to imply any linguistic deprivation in any accepted sense of that term on the part of such children. On the contrary, their linguistic experiences may be richer than many of their peers. However, the necessity to accommodate to English as a second language, or to a form of English different from their own, may impose additional problems and therefore increased vulnerability.

Worst of all, the children of ethnic minority groups grow up in a society which all too frequently rejects them in diverse ways, and in which unemployment strikes them particularly hard.

MULTIPLE DISADVANTAGE

The most 'vulnerable' children suffer from a multiplicity of social, emotional and economic disadvantages. These often inter-act and exert their influence from birth, or even before. The search for remedies has had limited success; attempts to apply them have been half-hearted, costly, and largely ineffective. Early prevention – chiefly in terms of supporting vulnerable parents – may well be the best policy. 'Preventative work undertaken with under-fives and their families can reduce the waste of expensive resources at a later stage, when the need to cope with the consequences of family stress and breakdown becomes more apparent and urgent' (C.P.R.S., 1978).

7. Concluding Thoughts and Unanswered Questions

A willingness to devote adequate resources to the care of children is the hallmark of a civilised society as well as an investment in our future. Some argue that we do not know enough to provide positive care and creative education for all children; others object that child rearing is essentially a personal, private matter; while yet others retort that we cannot afford to spend more. So A. E. Housman's despairing appeal 'When will I be dead and rid of the wrong my father did?' continues to be a reproach to our affluent society.

Granted that more needs to be found out about how best to promote children's all-round development, surely enough is known already to take action. If even half of what we now know were accepted with feeling and applied with understanding by all who have the care of children, then the revolution brought about in children's physical health in the past forty years might well be matched by a similar change in their psychological well-being. By strengthening their emotional resilience and increasing their capacity for learning, they would be better prepared to adapt to a rapidly changing world.

In what follows, I shall summarise my views on the needs of children; indicate some changes which are required in the climate of opinion about children's rights and parental responsibilities; and, finally, raise some questions to which answers must be sought.

THE NEEDS OF CHILDREN

There are four basic emotional needs which have to be met from the very beginning of life to enable a child to grow from helpless infancy to mature adulthood. These are: the need for love and security; for new experiences; for praise and recognition; and for responsibility. Their relative importance changes, of course, during the different stages of growth as do the ways in which they are met.

The need for love and security

Probably this is the most important because it provides the basis for all later relationships, not only within the family, but with friends, colleagues and eventually one's own family. On it depend the healthy development of the personality, the ability to care and respond to affection and, in time, to becoming a loving, caring parent. This need is met by the child experiencing from birth onwards a continuous, reliable, loving relationship – first, with his mother, then father and then an ever-widening circle of adults and contemporaries. The security of a familiar place and a known routine make for continuity and predictability in a world in which the child has to come to terms with so much that is new and changing. Also a stable family life provides him with a sense of personal continuity, of having a past as well as a future, and of a coherent and enduring identity.

The need for new experiences

Only if this need is adequately met throughout childhood and adolescence will a child's intelligence develop satisfactorily. Just as the body requires food for physical development and just as an appropriate balanced diet is essential for normal growth, so new experiences are needed for the mind. The most vital ingredients of this diet in early childhood are play and language. Through them, the child explores the world and learns to cope with it. This is as true for the objective outside world of reality as it is for the subjective internal world of thoughts and feelings.

New experiences facilitate the learning of one of the most important lessons of early life: learning how to learn; and learning that mastery brings joy and a sense of achievement. Educability depends not only on inborn capacity, but as much – if not more – on environmental opportunity and encouragement. The emotional and cultural climate of the home, as well as parental involvement and aspirations, can foster, limit or impair mental growth.

Play meets the need for new experiences in two major ways: it enables the child to learn about the world; and it provides a means of coping with and resolving conflicting emotions by allowing fantasy to over-ride reality and logic.

Probably the single and in the long run most crucial factor which promotes intellectual growth is the quality of the child's language environment: not merely how much he is talked to, but how relevant, distinctive and rich the conversation is. Language helps in learning to reason and to think, and also in making relationships.

Going to school is itself a major new experience which opens up a larger and more impersonal world. The child's progress will come to be powerfully affected by his teacher's attitudes, values and beliefs. Wide interests, enthusiasm for things of the mind and receptiveness to new ideas – all these are infectious. Teachers are in a powerful position to preserve, to awaken or to rekindle the curiosity and joy in learning about new things, shown by almost all young children.

The need for praise and recognition

To grow from a helpless infant into a self-reliant, self-accepting adult requires an immense amount of emotional, social and intellectual learning. It is accomplished by the child's modelling himself on the adults who are caring for him. The most effective incentives to bring this about – which requires a continuous effort, sustained throughout the years of growing up – are praise and recognition. Eventually, a job well done becomes its own reward but that is a very mature stage; and even the most mature adult responds, and indeed blossoms, when given occasionally some praise or other forms of recognition.

Because growing up is inevitably beset by difficulties, conflicts and setbacks, a strong incentive is needed. This is provided by the pleasure shown at success and the praise given to achievement by the adults who love the child and whom he in turn loves and wants to please. Encouragement and reasonable demands act as a spur to perseverance. The level of expectation is optimal when success is possible but not without effort. It cannot be the same for all children nor for all time. Rather, it must be geared to the individual child's capabilities at a given point in time and to the particular stage of his growth.

Teachers play a vital role too in meeting the need for praise and recognition; if for no other reason than because every child spends about half his waking life in school for at least eleven years. This provides an unrivalled opportunity to establish a favourable attitude to learning and also, where necessary, to improve or even rebuild the foundation for a child's self-esteem and hence his attitude to effort and achievement. To succeed in this task, a teacher must act on the assumption that every pupil has as yet unrealised potential for development which an appropriate 'diet' can call out, rather than accept past failures as indicating immutably limited learning ability.

The need for responsibility

This need is met by allowing the child to gain personal independence, at first through learning to look after himself in matters of his everyday care, such as feeding, dressing and washing himself. It is met too by his having possessions, however small and inexpensive, over which he is allowed to exercise absolute ownership. As he gets older, responsibility has to be extended to more important areas, ultimately allowing him freedom over his own actions. Eventually, in full maturity, he should be able to accept responsibility for others.

Granting increasing independence does not mean withholding one's views, tastes and choices, or the reasons for them; nor does it mean opting out from participating and guiding the lives of children; nor, indeed, condoning everything they do. On the contrary, children need a framework of guidance and of limits. They are helped by knowing what is expected or permitted, what the rules are, together with the reasons for them, and whether these are in their interests or in the interests of others.

How can responsibility be given to the immature and to the irresponsible? There is no way out of the dilemma that unless it is granted, the child cannot learn how to exercise it. Like every other skill, it needs to be practised under adult guidance which should gradually diminish. Training adolescents for responsibility is a particularly complex task. It requires a delicate balance between giving information and advice on the one hand and, on the other, leaving the making of decisions and coping with their consequences to the young person while yet being prepared to step in and help if things go badly wrong.

Schools have a vital contribution to make in this area. Those which emphasise cooperation rather than competition, which neither stream nor use corporal punishment have a lower incidence of bullying, violence and delinquency without any lowering of academic standards (Marjoribanks, 1978; Rutter et al., 1979).

Failure to meet children's needs

If one of the basic needs remains unmet, or is inadequately met, then development may become stunted or distorted. The consequences can be disastrous (and costly) later on, both for the individual and for society. Symptoms of maladjustment are, like pain, danger signals, indicating intolerable tension between the personality and the environment. The range of possible symptoms is wide but basically they fall into two broad categories: fight or flight, attack or withdrawal. Aggressiveness calls forth much stronger adult reactions whereas the timid, over-conforming child tends to be overlooked; yet both types of behaviour are equally significant calls for help, indicating that emotional, social or intellectual needs are not being adequately met.

Prisons, mental hospitals, borstals and schools for the maladjusted, contain a high proportion of individuals who in childhood were unloved and rejected. Their number is high too among the chronically unemployable and among able misfits. Anger, hate, lack of concern for others and an inability to make mutually satisfactory relationships are common reactions to having been unloved and rejected.

A child growing up in a discordant home is also liable to become emotionally disturbed or anti-social. A quarrelling, inadequate or disturbed parent makes a poor adult model. Parental hostility has a particularly harmful effect on a child's later development, especially on his ability to give, as an adult, unselfish loving care to his own children. Thus parental hostility perpetuates itself from one generation to another in what is literally an extremely vicious circle (Rutter and Madge, 1976).

If the need for new experiences is not adequately met throughout childhood and adolescence, then intellectual ability will remain stunted. Also, the more unstimulating, uneventful and dull life is, the more readily frustration, apathy, or restlessness set in. This is shown clearly by the contrast between the eagerness, alertness and vitality of normal toddlers whose life is filled with new experiences and challenges; and the aimlessness and boredom of adolescents with nothing to do and nowhere to go.

The urban environment is hostile to the young: there is little freedom or safety to explore or experiment, particularly without adult supervision. In seeking – legitimately – for the excitement of new experiences, where few are to be found or attainable, the forbidden, risky or dangerous are liable to acquire an aura of daring and excitement. What may start as a lark, giving vent to high spirits and the desire for adventure, can then all too easily turn into vandalism and mindless destruction.

Unfortunately, praise and recognition are almost invariably given for achievement rather than effort. In consequence, this need is most readily and often satisfied in the case of intelligent, healthy, adjusted and attractive children. In contrast, the intellectually slow, culturally disadvantaged, emotionally neglected or maladjusted get far less, if any, praise and recognition. Yet their need is immeasurably greater. Whatever small successes they achieve inevitably demand far more effort and perseverance; yet they receive less reward because they achieve less.

In school, praising for achievement instead of effort has very harmful effects on the slower learner as well as on the child with emotional or physical handicaps: he has no chance of shining and always finds himself near the bottom of his class. Such constant failure inevitably damages self-esteem and motivation. The teacher who believes that what matters most is the effort a child makes, and who praises whenever there is improvement however slow and limited, provides an appropriate incentive for all pupils, whatever their abilities. For better or for worse, the encouragement and expectations of parents and teachers have a most powerful influence on a child's progress.

There is controversy between those who demand equal educational opportunity for all; those who advocate that special attention ought to be devoted to the abler child; and those who argue that positive discrimination must be exercised in favour of the less able and under-privileged. The conflict between these viewpoints is, however, more apparent than real. It springs from the mistaken belief that all men are equal despite the enormous disparity in physical, intellectual and creative potential found in all walks of life. Equality of opportunity is the right of every child. To expect equal capacity to make use of this opportunity runs counter to common sense and experience.

Instead, we must act as if all children were equal and then respect, as well as accept and cater for, their differences. Within such a framework, it is legitimate both to provide a democracy of opportunity while at the same time to strive for excellence so as to ensure an aristocracy of achievement.

When the fourth basic emotional need, namely to exercise responsibility, is denied opportunities for fulfilment, then the child will fail to develop a sense of responsibility for himself, for others or for material objects. When such denial has gone hand in hand with a lack of training in self-control and in planning ahead, then such youngsters will tend to be impulsive, unwilling to wait and work for what they want, contemptuous of the rights of others – in short, irresponsible. A high proportion of the self-same young people will on leaving school find themselves in jobs which give them little, if any, responsibility. Work which fails to fulfil the need for involvement is likely to heighten the sense of alienation and rejection. Feeling that society has disowned them may well engender a feeling that they in turn owe nothing to society.

The cost of prevention

How costly would it be to ensure that children's needs are met, so as to promote and ensure their optimal emotional, social, intellectual and educational development? No one really knows because no serious consideration has been given to this question. How much would it cost to have supportive services available to the family, sufficient in quality and quantity, to prevent children who are 'vulnerable' or 'at risk' growing up emotionally disturbed, socially deviant, intellectually stunted and educationally backward? Again, no one can really say because the question has not been asked.

Nevertheless, some argue that as a society we simply cannot afford to pay either for wide-ranging preventive services or for comprehensive rehabilitation and treatment facilities. Is this not fallacious? Surely the question is: can we afford not to do so? Failure to provide the necessary programmes for children and their families merely postpones the day when the community has to pay the much higher price for not willing the means earlier. The cost in the long run is extremely high: not only in terms of human misery and wasted potentialities but also in terms of unemployability, mental ill health, crime and a renewed cycle of inadequate parenting. Even in the short run, it is by no means economic to do too little and to do it too late.

For example, in most cases, emotional, social or learning difficulties come to light when a child starts school. Inevitably, providing special classes, school psychological or psychiatric services is costly; but if the child's difficulties are so severe or his family background so unsatisfactory that residential facilities are required, then the cost is ten times as high (Pond and Arie, 1971). Moreover, because there are not enough trained personnel in any of the helping professions – whether remedial teachers, social workers, psychologists, psychiatrists or speech therapists – waiting lists are long and only those whose needs are the most urgent have any hope of receiving special help early. The later it is given, the more difficult and lengthy, and hence the more costly, the treatment and the less hopeful the prognosis. So in the event we may well be paying the most for the least effective intervention simply because prevention is not only better but cheaper than cure (Pringle, 1980).

TODAY'S CHILDREN – TOMORROW'S PARENTS

Children inevitably depend on others for their well-being, care and education; they have no vote or voice in the running of the community, either at local or national level; and resources devoted to them are society's investment in tomorrow's parents. For all practical purposes of social policy, we must act on the assumption that the environment is of over-riding importance and that the early years of life are particularly vital. To develop the potential for becoming human, the baby must needs have a human environment; and the most efficient and economical system known to man for making human infants human is the family. Hence a long-term policy for children must be based on improving the quality of family care and of education from cradle through adulthood. To do so requires two wide-ranging changes: a different attitude to parenthood and child rearing; and a willingness to provide more adequate services for families and children, if only for the sake of the latter. The implication of the first change is discussed in this section.

Children's rights and parental responsibilities

The prevailing climate of opinion must be changed in a number of respects. First, children's rights and parental responsibilities need to be re-defined. Current attitudes on the paramountcy of 'biological' parenthood are ambivalent and contradictory. Both in law and in practice we often act as if the blood tie and 'natural' parenthood necessarily ensured satisfactory parenting. Yet we fail to provide sufficient community support to enable a child to be looked after by his own family at times of difficulty (say mother's illness or pregnancy); in consequence, thousands of pre-school children come into public care every year.

Furthermore, we so over-value the child's ties with his natural parents that we are far too slow to consider severing them permanently when the parents are disturbed or rejecting, even to a pathological degree. Thus some babies who have been brutally assaulted are returned to their homes when both common sense and clinical evidence indicate that there is a high chance of it happening again with the risk of permanent injury or death (Pringle, 1981). Similarly, this misplaced faith in the blood tie, and an unjustified optimism about the chances of successfully awakening or rekindling parental interest when a child has been to all intents and purposes abandoned, condemns thousands of them to remain in long-term public care without permanent substitute parents.

Secondly, the current over-romanticised picture of parenthood, and of motherhood in particular – projected by the media and the advertising industry – ought to be changed. A more realistic and perhaps even daunting awareness needs to be created of the arduous demands which child rearing makes on the emotions, energy, time and finances, as well as of the inevitable constraints on personal independence, freedom of movement and, indeed, one's whole way of life. Babies should be presented 'truthfully', warts and all – sometimes fretful and demanding, often wet, smelly, crying at night and 'unreasonable' – rather than with a permanent angelic, dimply smile and sunny temper. Deglamourising parenthood in this way will not deter those who truly want to care for children but it may act as a brake on those with unrealistic expectations.

Thirdly, several other notions, which have no foundation in fact, should also be dispelled: that having a child is the sole or most important or easiest way to feminine fulfilment; that a baby completes a home, rather like a T.V. set or fridge; that it will cement an unsatisfactory or failing marriage; that maternity has a therapeutic effect, particularly on girls who were themselves rejected in childhood; that a child belongs to his parents like their other possessions; and that he should be grateful to his parents even though he did not ask to be born.

Responsible parenthood

The myth of the blood tie should be replaced by the concept of responsible and informed parenthood. The ability and willingness to undertake its responsibilities are neither dependent nor necessarily consequent upon, biological parenthood. Rather it is the unconditional desire to provide a caring home, together with the emotional maturity to do so, which are the hallmarks of good parenting. Responsible parenthood also includes having only as many children as a couple can emotionally cope with and financially afford.

Common sense suggests that very young parents, themselves not yet fully mature emotionally, are less able to provide the emotional support so vital to a child's optimal development. Being at the beginning of their working life, financial and housing problems are likely to be additional difficulties. But perhaps one of the main reasons why the rate of marriage failure is highest among those who marry young is the fact that neither partner has as yet reached his mature level of emotional, social and intellectual development. When the pace of this growth is markedly different for one spouse, then the couple will later on be no longer as well-matched as they had been. It would be in the long-term interest both of the future parents and of their children if parenthood were postponed until both partners are fully mature emotionally. For this to happen, a social climate will have to be created in which it is considered irresponsible to have children before, say, the age of twenty-two or twenty-three (Whitehead, 1977).

Preparation for parenthood, including family planning, could make an important contribution. Modern parenthood is too demanding and complex a task to be performed well merely because we all have once been children ourselves. Those who have been deprived of adequate parental care, thus not having had an opportunity to observe even those parental skills which were practised a generation ago, have little chance of becoming in turn responsible parents themselves.

An effective programme of preparation for parenthood would have to adopt a wide and comprehensive base. It should deal with the whole area of human relations and in particular with child development; first-hand experience of babies and young children should be an essential part of the programme; as should be an understanding of the ways in which the relations between a married couple are bound to change when they become parents. These changes are emotional since loving and caring has now to be shared with a totally dependent, demanding new-comer; they are social in that child-rearing curtails the personal freedom, leisure time and activities of both parents; and financial since families with very young children are likely to be at the lowest earning point of their working lives. Significantly, the need for a wide programme of preparation for parenthood is well appreciated by young people themselves (Fogelman, 1976).

Responsible parenthood must come to mean that the parental life style has been freely and deliberately chosen in the full realisation of its demands, constraints, satisfactions and challenges. Since the technological know-how is also now available it would be possible to translate into reality the slogan 'every child a wanted child'. Then there would be a much better chance than at present that the needs of children will be met. How to do so has been summarised in the following ten child care commandments. These are based on what has been said in Chapters 1, 2 and 3.

The art of child-rearing

These ten child care commandments are rather in the nature of guidelines. Inevitably only a few generalisations can ever be of universal application because of the uniqueness of each individual – father, mother and child; and for this reason the relationships between the parents themselves, and between them and each child, are also unique. A parent's best guide is his own quality of understanding, combined with his knowledge of developmental needs, both of which are then applied to the upbringing of each individual child. An understanding of a child's physical and mental abilities at any given stage, and hence his readiness at a given time to respond and adapt, is the most reliable gauge of whether parental expectations are appropriate.

It is an illusory, and sometimes even harmful, aim to treat each child alike. What is needed is a 'tailor-made' approach fashioned to suit each child but based on the general principles of child-rearing embodied in the ten child care commandments. Only by allowing for individual differences can we ensure an appropriate environment for each member of a family. In this way too we shall avoid trying to fashion a child in our own image and so avoid disappointment for ourselves and a sense of inadequacy in our children.

Ten Child Care Commandments

1 Give continuous, consistent, loving care – it's as essential for the mind's health as food is for the body.
2 Give generously of your time and understanding – playing with and reading to your child matters more than a tidy, smooth-running home.
3 Provide new experiences and bathe your child in language from birth onwards – they enrich his growing mind.
4 Encourage him to play in every way both by himself and with other children – exploring, imitating, constructing, pretending and creating.
5 Give more praise for effort than for achievement.
6 Give him ever-increasing responsibility – like all skills, it needs to be practised.
7 Remember that every child is unique – so suitable handling for one may not be right for another.
8 Make the way you show disapproval fit your child's temperament, age and understanding.
9 Never threaten that you will stop loving him or give him away; you may reject his behaviour but never suggest that you might reject him.
10 Don't expect gratitude; your child did not ask to be born – the choice was yours.

SOME UNANSWERED QUESTIONS

1 To begin with, should we ask the question: into what kind of people do we want today's children to grow? How it is answered materially affects child-rearing methods.

2 Should there be two different forms of marriage? One would involve only a simple contract – designed to protect the interests of both partners in case of a break-down – which could be readily terminated at the request of either. The other contract would involve a much more binding commitment of at least ten or fifteen years because the couple were wishing to raise a family and were prepared to put the needs of their children for stability and continuous, loving care above their own individual self-fulfilment; this contract would be much more difficult to terminate. In consequence the

American trend towards 'serial marriages' would then become the prerogative only of the childless by choice.

3 Why do we assume that the light of nature is sufficient for parents to know what the needs of children are and how these are best met? Is it because we have all once been children and learned from the child-rearing practices of our own parents? Yet most people would not accept the similar argument that because we have all been to school we could be adequate teachers without any training; in fact, professional teacher training has become longer to keep pace with increasing knowledge.

4 What methods and what settings would be most effective for the dissemination of knowledge and understanding of children's needs? And should current as well as new initiatives and schemes be monitored and evaluated to enable guidelines to be developed for future use?

5 Is it sensible for religious education to remain the only subject which schools must provide in our secularist, multi-denominational society? Is there not a stronger case for making preparation for parenthood a required subject at least in all secondary schools since the vast majority of pupils are likely to become parents? Presenting a balanced, honest picture of parenthood could contribute to their making a more informed, responsible choice of life style later on. Also might its status be raised if a more general understanding were brought about of why it is among the world's most important, creative and difficult jobs, if done well?

6 What are the most effective ways of supporting and supplementing parental care at different ages and stages? How can maternal involvement in services for pre-school children be maximised on the one hand; yet on the other hand, how can she be provided with occasional but regular relief from the taxing daily task of caring for very young children? By what means might the energies of the young and the elderly in the neighbourhood be harnessed for that purpose?

7 How can the rights of children, particularly the very young, be safeguarded when they are subtly but insistently and dangerously, being undermined by the women's movement, aided and abetted by the media? While a woman certainly should have the right not to become a mother, the current dogma that 'a baby should not be

allowed to make any difference to a woman's life' is not only double-think but also ignores the basic needs of young children.

8 Should cost benefit studies be undertaken of providing sufficiently generous allowances to enable one parent (including a single parent) to look after young children full-time? And to establish how many mothers (or fathers) would wish during these earliest years to exercise this option in preference to an outside paid job?

9 Do we go too far in asserting that the way parents bring up their children is solely their own concern? Need a new balance be struck between parental rights and parental responsibilities? The great majority do, of course, give loving, concerned, responsible care. But what about the minority who are not able or willing to do so? Can children be compensated for ineffective or harmful parental handling? And if it is so damaging that a substitute family is the only solution to safeguard a child's long-term development, what preparation is necessary to ensure the success of this transplant operation?

10 What are the qualities, circumstances or relationships which enable a child from a grossly impoverished, depriving or neglectful home to emerge nevertheless apparently unscathed? A great deal is known now about the harmful effects of impaired family relations, emotional deprivation and intellectual under-stimulation. Yet some children manage to triumph over appalling odds. Gaining a better understanding of the mechanisms at work would surely aid prevention and possibly rehabilitation, too?

11 Why have we for so long neglected one of the most important tools of prevention, namely listening to the voices of children themselves? Long before they can speak, infants reveal by their behaviour and through their play whether their need for loving, consistent care is being met or not; while older children show even more unmistakably 'early warning' signs and, of course, can express their anxieties verbally, provided there is someone who is perceptive enough and has time enough to listen.

12 If prevention is to become a reality, is there perhaps a need for an 'objective watch-dog' whose brief it is to be exclusively concerned for the well-being of children across central government and local government departments; across professional disciplines; and across

all relevant services including legal and housing provision? Might either a Minister for Children who has no departmental responsibilities, rather on the model of our Minister for the Disabled, or an Ombudsman, along the lines adopted in Sweden, help to focus attention on the needs of children amid the clamour from the many competing interests of a wide variety of pressure groups for adults? After five years work the Swedish Ombudsman concluded that 'even in a country with a very wide-ranging social service system, there are many fields in which the interests of the child are not met or protected.' Much suffering and stunting and much long-term damage to children's potentialities could be avoided by the greater protection afforded them earlier on by some such agency.

To make man more perfect in body and mind has been an age-old dream. In the physical realm the prospect of positive good health is becoming a reality within reach of at least the developed countries. 'The developed, integrated human personality is without question the highest thing we know in the universe.' (Sir Julian Huxley.) Are we now reaching a cross-road? Given the will and willing the resources, science and technology may be able to provide the knowledge and to develop the techniques to bring the second part of man's dream of perfectibility at least within the realm of possibility. A compassionate society in which individual fulfilment and freedom are reconciled with the individual's obligations and commitment to the needs of his community – can there be a higher stake, a more worthwhile goal or a more exciting challenge than improving in this way the quality of life for all our children?

References

ALLAND, A. (1972). *The Human Imperative*, Columbia University Press, New York.

ALLEN, F. H. and PEARSON, G. H. J. (1928). The emotional problems of the physically handicapped child. *British Journal of Medical Psychology*, **8** (3), 212–35.

AMBROSE, J. A. (1963). The concept of a critical period for the development of social responsiveness in early human infancy. *Determinants of Infant Behaviour*, B. Foss (ed.), vol. 2. Methuen.

AMBROSE, J. A. (ed.) (1970). *Stimulation in Early Infancy*, Academic Press, New York.

ANDERSON, R. H. and SHANE, H. G. (1971). *As the Twig is Bent*, Houghton, Mifflin & Co., Boston.

ANDRY, R. G. (1960). *Delinquency and Parental Pathology*, Methuen.

ARGYLE, M. (1969). *Social Interaction*, Methuen.

ARIÈS, P. (1962). *Centuries of Childhood*, Jonathan Cape.

AVGAR, A., BRONFENBRENNER, U. and HENDERSON, C. R. (1977). Socialization practices of parents, teachers and peers in Israel: kibbutz, moshav and city. *Child Development*, **48** 1219–27.

BANKS, O. and FINLAYSON, D. (1973). *Success and Failure in the Secondary School: an interdisciplinary approach*, Methuen.

BARATZ, S. S. and BARATZ, J. C. (1970). Early childhood intervention: the social science base of institutional racism. *Harvard Educational Review*, **40** (1), 29–50.

BARTEN, S. S. and BLANK, M. (1971). Soviet research on speech and language: an American perspective. *Early Child Development*, **1** (1), 3–14.

BARNES, D., BRITTON, J. and ROSEN, H. (1971). *Language, the Learner and the School*, Penguin.

BAYLEY, N. (1964). Consistency of maternal and child behaviors in the Berkeley Growth Study. *Vita Humana*, **7** (2), 73–95.

BELL, R. Q. (1968). A re-interpretation of the direction of effects in studies of socialisation, *Psychological Review*, **75** (1), 81–95.

BELSON, W. A. (1975). *Juvenile Theft: The Causal Factors*, Harper and Row.

BENN, C. (1969). Marriage breakdown and the individual. *Divorce, Society and the Law*, H. A. Finlay (ed.), Butterworth and Co., New South Wales, Australia.

BENTHALL, J. (ed.) (1973). *The Limits of Human Nature*, Allen Lane, The Penguin Press.

BERGER, M. and PASSINGHAM, R. E. (1972). Early experience and other environmental factors: an overview. *Handbook of Abnormal Psychology*, H. J. Eysenck (ed.), 2nd ed., Pitman.

BERLIN, I. N. (ed.) (1975). *Advocacy for Child Mental Health*: Brunner/Mazel, New York.

BERLYNE, D. E. (1960). *Conflict, Arousal and Curiosity*, McGraw-Hill, New York.

BERNSTEIN, B. (1961a). Social structure, language and learning. *Educational Research*, **3** (2), 163–76.

BERNSTEIN, B. (1961b). Aspects of language and learning in the genesis of the social process. *Journal of Child Psychology and Psychiatry*, **1** (4), 313–24.

BERNSTEIN, B. (ed.) (1973). Applied studies towards a sociology of language. *Class, Codes and Control*, vol. 2. Routledge and Kegan Paul.

BERNSTEIN, B. (1977). Theoretical studies towards a sociology of language. *Class, Codes and Control*, vol. 1, 2nd ed., Routledge and Kegan Paul.

BERRIDGE, D. (1985) *Children's Homes*. Blackwell.

BERRY, J. (1972). *Social Work with Children*, Routledge and Kegan Paul.

BIRCH, H. and GUSSOW, J. (1970). *Disadvantaged Children: Health, Nutrition and School Failure*, Harcourt, Brace and World, New York.

BIRLEY, J. L. T. (1973). The effect of the environment on the individual. *Proceedings of the Royal Society of Medicine*, **66** (1, part 2), 93–8.

BLANK, M. and SOLOMON, F. (1969). How shall the disadvantaged be taught? *Child Development*, **49** (1), 47–61.

BLOOM, B. S. (1964). *Stability and Change in Human Characteristics*, John Wiley, New York.

BLOOM, B. S. (1974). Affective consequences of school achievement. *Advances in Educational Psychology*, M. L. Kellmer Pringle and V. P. Varma (eds.), vol. 2. University of London Press.

BLOOM, B. S., DAVIES, A. and HESS, R. (1965). *Compensatory Education for Cultural Deprivation*. Holt, Rinehart and Winston, New York.

BOHMAN, M. (1971). A comparative study of adopted children, foster children and children in their biological environment born after undesired pregnancies. *Acta Paediatrica Scandinavica*, Suppl. 221.

BOHMAN, M. and SIGVARDSSON, S. (1985). A prospective longitudinal study of adoption. *Longitudinal Studies in Child Psychology and Psychiatry*, A. R. Nicol (ed.), John Wiley, New York.

BOWLBY, J. (1951). *Maternal Care and Mental Health*. World Health Organisation, Geneva.

BOWLBY, J. (1969). Attachment. *Attachment and Loss*, **1**. Hogarth Press.

BOWLBY, J. (1979). *The Making and Breaking of Affectional Bonds*. Tavistock.

BOWLBY, J. (1982). Attachment and loss: Retrospect and prospect.

American Journal of Orthopsychiatry, **52** (4), 664–78.

BOWLBY, J. and PARKES, C. D. (1970). Separation and loss within the family. *The Child in his Family*, E. J. Anthony and C. M. Koupernik (eds.), John Wiley, New York.

BRIERLEY, J. (1976). *The Growing Brain*, N.F.E.R., Slough.

BRONFENBRENNER, U. (1967). The psychological costs of quality and equality in education. *Child Development*, **38** (3), 909–25.

BRONFENBRENNER, U. (1968). Early deprivation in mammals and man: a cross-species analysis. *Early Experience and Behavior*, G. Newton and S. Levine (eds.), C. C. Thomas, Springfield, Ill.

BRONFENBRENNER, U. (1970). *Two Worlds of Childhood: U.S. and U.S.S.R.* Russell Sage Foundation, New York.

BRONFENBRENNER, U. (1973). Developmental research, public policy and the ecology of childhood. Paper read at the Annual Meeting of the Society for Research in Child Development. Philadelphia, 31 March.

BROPHY, J. E. (1983). Research on the self-fulfilling prophecy and teacher expectations. *Journal of Educational Psychology*, **75** (5), 631–61.

BROWN, C. (1954). *My Left Foot*. Secker and Warburg.

BRUNER, J. S. et al. (1966). *Studies in Cognitive Growth*. John Wiley, New York.

BURT, SIR C. (1975). *The Gifted Child*. Hodder and Stoughton.

BURT, SIR C.(1977). *The Subnormal Mind*, 3rd ed., Oxford.

BUTLER, N. R. and ALBERMAN, E. (eds.) (1969). *Perinatal Problems*. Livingstone.

BUTLER, N. R. and BONHAM, G. H. (1963). *Perinatal Mortality*. Livingstone.

BUTLER, N. R. and GOLDSTEIN, H. (1973). Smoking in pregnancy and subsequent child development. *British Medical Journal*, 8 Dec., **4**, 573–5.

CALDWELL, B. M. (1970). The effects of psychosocial deprivation on human development in infancy. *Merrill-Palmer Quarterly*, **16** (3), 260–77.

CAMPBELL, D. (1972). Activity and attachment in early life. *Proceedings of the British Psychological Society*, London Conference.

CARLSON, E. R. (1952). *Born that Way*. Arthur James.

CARNEGIE UNITED KINGDOM TRUST. (1964). *Handicapped Children and their Families*. Dunfermline, Scotland.

CENTRAL POLICY REVIEW STAFF. (1978). *Services for young children with working mothers*: H.M.S.O.

CENTRAL STATISTICAL OFFICE. (1986). *Social Trends* (16). H.M.S.O.

CHAZAN, M. (1963). Maladjustment, attainment and sociometric status. *University College of Education Journal*, 4–7.

CHAZAN, M., LAING, A. and JACKSON, S. (1971). *Just before School*. Blackwell, Oxford.

CHAZAN, M., LAING, A., BAILEY, M. S. and JONES, G. (1980). *Some of our Children*. Open Books.

CHIBUCOS, T. and KAIL, P. (1981). Longitudinal examination of father–infant interaction and infant–father interaction. *Merrill-Palmer Quarterly*, **27**, 81–96.

CHILD POVERTY ACTION GROUP. (1984). *Poverty: What Poverty?*

CLARKE, A. D. B. and CLARKE, A. M. (1972). Consistency and variability in the growth of human characteristics. *Advances in Educational Psychology*, **1**, W. D. Wall and V. P Varma (eds.), University of London Press.

CLARKE, A. D. B. and CLARKE, A. M. (1978). *Readings from Mental Deficiency: The Changing Outlook*. Methuen.

COHEN, LORD OF BIRKENHEAD. (1965). Foreword to *Investment in Children*. M. L. Kellmer Pringle (ed.), Longman.

COLEMAN, J. S. et al. (1966). *Equality of Educational Opportunity*. U.S. Government Printing Office, Washington D.C.

COOKSEY, G. (1972). Teachers, parents and the social services. *The Challenge of Change*, M. Kogan and M. Pope (eds.), N.F.E.R., Slough, for National Children's Bureau.

COONS, J. and SUGARMAN, S. (1978). *Education by Choice: the Case for Family Control*. University of California Press.

COOPER, J. (1969). Group treatment in residential care. *Caring for Children*, M. L. Kellmer Pringle (ed.), Longman in association with the National Children's Bureau.

COOPER, J. (1978). *Patterns of Family Placement: Current Issues in Fostering and Adoption*. National Children's Bureau.

CORNISH, D. B. and CLARKE, R. V. G. (1975). *Residential Treatment and Its Effects on Delinquency*. Home Office Research Study, H.M.S.O.

CREBER, J. W. P. (1972). *Lost for Words*. Penguin.

CREIGHTON, S. J. (1984). *Trends in Child Abuse 1977–1982*. National Society for the Prevention of Cruelty to Children.

CRELLIN, E., PRINGLE, M. L. K. and WEST, P. (1971). *Born Illegitimate*. N.F.E.R., Slough, for National Children's Bureau.

DALLY, A. (1976). *Mothers: their Power and Influence*. Weidenfeld and Nicholson.

DARLINGTON, R. B. (1980). Pre-school programmes and later school competence of children from low-income families. *Science*, **208**, 202.

DAVIE, R. (1972). The behaviour and adjustment in school of seven-year-olds; sex and social class differences. *Early Child Development and Care*, **2** (1), 39–47.

DAVIE, R. (1973). Eleven years of childhood. *Statistical News* (22), 14–18.

DAVIE, R., BUTLER, N. and GOLDSTEIN, H. (1972). *From Birth to Seven*. Longman in association with the National Children's Bureau.

DAVIES, B. (1969). Non-swinging youth. *New Society*, 3 July, **14** (353), 8–10.

DAVIS, K. (1947). Final note on a case of extreme isolation. *American Journal of Sociology*, **52** (5), 432–7.

DE BONO, E. (1972). *Children Solve Problems*. Allen Lane.

DENENBERG, V. H. (1969). Animal studies of early experience: some principles which have implications for human development. *Minnesota Symposium in Child Psychology*, **3**, J. P. Hill (ed.), University of Minnesota Press.

DEPARTMENT OF EDUCATION AND SCIENCE (1985). *Education for All. The Report of the Committee of Enquiry into the Education of Children from Ethnic Minority Groups. (Swann Report)*. H.M.S.O.

DEPARTMENT OF THE ENVIRONMENT. (1973). Children at play. *Design Bulletin* (27), H.M.S.O.

DEPARTMENT OF HEALTH AND SOCIAL SECURITY. (1972). *The 'Battered Baby' Syndrome; an analysis of reports submitted by Medical Officers of Health and Children's Officers*. H.M.S.O.

DEPARTMENT OF HEALTH AND SOCIAL SECURITY. (1981). *A Study of the Boarding out of Children*. H.M.S.O.

DEPARTMENT OF HEALTH AND SOCIAL SECURITY. (1982). *Child Abuse*. H.M.S.O.

DEPARTMENT OF HEALTH AND SOCIAL SECURITY. (1985). *Social Work Decisions in Child Care*. H.M.S.O.

DEVEREUX, E. C., BRONFENBRENNER, U. and RODGERS, R. R. (1969). Child rearing in England and the United States: a cross-national comparison. *Journal of Marriage and the Family*, **31** (2), 257–70.

DINNAGE, R. (1971). The Handicapped Child. *Research Review*, **1**: *Neurological Handicaps*. Longman in association with the National Children's Bureau.

DINNAGE, R. (1972). The Handicapped Child. *Research Review*, **2**: *Sensory and Physical Handicaps*. Longman in association with the National Children's Bureau.

DINNAGE, R. (1986a). *The Child with a Chronic Medical Problem: An Annotated Bibliography*. N.F.E.R., Slough for National Children's Bureau.

DINNAGE, R. (1986b). *The Child with Spina Bifida: An Annotated Bibliography*. N.F.E.R., Slough, for National Children's Bureau.

DINNAGE, R. (1986c). *The Child with Cerebral Palsy: An Annotated Bibliography*. N.F.E.R., Slough, for National Children's Bureau.

DINNAGE, R. (1986d). *The Orthopaedically Handicapped Child: An Annotated Bibliography*. N.F.E.R., Slough, for National Children's Bureau.

DINNAGE, R. (1986e). *The Child with Epilepsy: An Annotated Bibliography*. N.F.E.R., Slough, for National Children's Bureau.

DINNAGE, R. and GOOCH, S. (1986f). *The Child with Asthma: An Annotated Bibliography*. N.F.E.R., Slough, for National Children's Bureau.

DINNAGE, R. and PRINGLE, M. L. KELLMER. (1967a). *Foster Care – Facts and Fallacies*. Longman in association with the National Children's Bureau.

DINNAGE, R. and PRINGLE, M. L. KELLMER. (1967b). *Residential Care – Facts and Fallacies*. Longman in association with the National

Children's Bureau.

DOBBING, J. and SMART, J. L. (1973). Early under-nutrition, brain development and behaviour. *Ethology and Development*. S. A. Barnett (ed.), Spastics Society and Heinemann.

DONNISON, D. (ed.) (1972). *A Pattern of Disadvantage*, N.F.E.R., Slough, for National Children's Bureau.

DOUGLAS, J. W. B. (1964). *The Home and the School*. MacGibbon and Kee.

DOUGLAS, J. W. B. (1970). Broken families and child behaviour. *Journal of Royal College of Physicians*, **4** (3), 203–10.

DOUGLAS, J. W. B., ROSS, J. M. and SIMPSON, H. R. (1968). *All Our Future*. Peter Davies.

DOWDALL, C. B. and COLANGELO, N. (1982). Underachieving gifted students: Review and implications. *Gifted Child Quarterly* (26), 179–84.

DUNLOP, A. B. (1975). Experience of residential treatment and its effectiveness. *Home Office Research Unit: Research Bulletin*, **2**, 22–5.

EARECKSON, J. (1978). *Joni*. Pickering and Inglis.

EIBL-EIBESFELDT, I. (1967). Concepts of ethology and their significance in the study of human behavior. *Early Behavior: Comparative and Developmental Approaches*. H. Stevenson, E. Hess and H. Rheingold (eds.), John Wiley, New York.

ENTWISTLE, H. (1978). *Class, Culture and Education*. Methuen.

ESSEN, J. (1978). Living in one-parent families: income and expenditure. *Poverty*, **40** (23).

ESSEN, J. (1979). Living in one-parent families: attainment at school. *Child: Care, Health and Development*, **5** (3), 83–93.

ESSEN, J., LAMBERT, L. and HEAD, J. (1976). School attainment of children who have been in care. *Child: Care, Health and Development*, **2** (6), 339–51.

ESSEN, J. and WEDGE, P. (1982). *Continuities in Childhood Disadvantage*. Heinemann Educational Books.

EYSENCK, H. (1984). Recent advances in the theory and measurement of intelligence. *Early Child Development and Care*, **15** (2–3), 97–116.

EYSENCK, H. J. and KAMIN, L. J. (1981). *Intelligence: The Battle for the Mind*. Pan Books.

FANSHEL, D. and SHINN, E. B. (1978). *Children in Foster Care: a Longitudinal Investigation*. Columbia University Press, New York.

FERRI, E. (1976). *Growing Up in a One Parent Family*. N.F.E.R., Slough, for National Children's Bureau.

FERRI, E. (1984). *Stepchildren: A National Study*. N.F.E.R., Slough.

FERRI, E. and ROBINSON, H. (1976). *Coping Alone*. N.F.E.R., Slough, for National Children's Bureau.

FITZHERBERT, K. (1977). *Child Care Services and the Teacher*. Temple Smith.

FLAVELL, J. H. (1963). *Developmental Psychology of Jean Piaget*. Van Nostrand, Princeton, N.J.

FOGELMAN, K. (ed.) (1976). *Britain's Sixteen Year Olds*. National Children's Bureau.

FOGELMAN, K. (ed.) (1983). *Growing Up in Great Britain*. Macmillan for the National Children's Bureau.

FOGELMAN, K. and GOLDSTEIN, H. (1976). Social factors associated with changes in educational attainment between 7 and 11 years of age. *Educational Studies*, **2**, 95–109.

FOGELMAN, K. and GORBACH, P. (1978). Age of starting school and attainment at 11. *Educational Research*, **21** (1).

FORSSMAN, H. and THUWE, I. (1965). One hundred and twenty children born after application for therapeutic abortion was refused. *Acta Pyschiatrica Scandinavia*, **42** (4), 71–88.

FRANKLIN, A. WHITE (1977a). *The Challenge of Child Abuse*. Academic Press.

FRANKLIN, A. WHITE (1977b). *Child Abuse: Prediction, Prevention and Follow up*. Churchill Livingstone.

GEORGE, V. (1970). *Foster Care: Theory and Practice*. Routledge and Kegan Paul.

GEORGE, V. and WILDING, P. (1972). *Motherless Families*. Routledge and Kegan Paul.

GEWIRTZ, H. B. and GEWIRTZ, J. L. (1969). Caretaking settings, background events and behaviour differences in four Israeli child rearing environments: some preliminary trends. *Determinants of Behaviour*, **4**, B. M. Foss (ed.), Methuen.

GIBSON, J. (1969). The mentally retarded child in hospital. Suggestions for improving care and stimulation. *Clinical Pediatrics*, **8** (5), 256–7.

GIL, D. (1971). *Violence against Children*. Harvard University Press, Cambridge, Mass.

GLUECK, S. and GLUECK, E. T. (1962). *Family Environment and Delinquency*. Kegan Paul.

GOLDBERG, S. (1983). Parent–infant bonding: another look. *Child Development*, **54** (6), 1355–82.

GOLDFARB, W. (1943). The effects of early institutional care on adolescent personality. *Journal of Experimental Education*, **12** (2), 108–29.

GOLDSTEIN, J., FREUD, A. and SOLNIT, A. J. (1980). *Beyond the Best Interests of the Child*. Burnett Books.

GOOCH, S. and PRINGLE, M. L. KELLMER. (1966). *Four Years On*. Longman in association with the National Children's Bureau.

GRAY, P. H. (1958). Theory and evidence of imprinting in human infants. *Journal of Psychology*, **46** (2), 155–66.

HALSEY, A. H. (1973). E.P.A. Problems and Policies. *Educational priority*, **1**, H.M.S.O.

HAMILL, L. (1979). Wives as sole and joint breadwinners. *Government Economic Service Working Paper*, **13** D.H.S.S.

HAMPSON, J. L. and HAMPSON, J. G. (1961). The entogenesis of sexual behavior in man. *Sex and Internal Secretions*, chap. 23, 1401–32. W. C. Young (ed.), Baillière, Tindall and Cox.

HARLOW, H. F. and GRIFFIN, G. (1965). Induced mental and social deficits in rhesus monkeys. *The Biosocial Basis of Mental Retardation*, S. F. Osler and R. E. Cooke (eds.), John Hopkins Press.

HARLOW, H. F. and HARLOW, M. K. (1969). Effects of various mother–infant relationships on rhesus monkey behaviour. *Determinants of Infant Behaviour*, **4**, 15–36, B. M. Foss (ed.), Methuen.

HARLOW, H. F. and HARLOW, M. K. (1970). Developmental aspects of emotional behavior. *Physiological Correlates of Emotion*, P. Black (ed.), Academic Press.

HELFER, R. E. and KEMPE, C. H. (eds.) (1968). *The Battered Child*. University of Chicago Press.

HELFER, R. E. and KEMPE, C. H. (eds.) (1971). *Helping the Battered Child and his Family*. University of Chicago Press.

HEMMING, J. (1974). Emotional and moral aspects of adolescence. *Advances in Educational Psychology*, **2** chap. 15, M. L. Kellmer Pringle and V. P. Varma (eds.), University of London Press.

HERBERT, M., SLUCKIN, W. and SLUCKIN, A. (1982). Mother-to-infant bonding. *Journal of Child Psychology and Psychiatry*, **23** (3), 205–21.

HESS, R. D. and SHIPMAN, V. C. (1965). Early experience and the socialization of cognitive modes in children. *Child Development*, **36** (4), 869–86.

HETHERINGTON, E. M., COX, M. and COX, R. (1982). Effects of divorce on parents and children. *Non-traditional Families*, M. Lamb (ed.), Erlbaum: Hillsdale, New Jersey.

HEWETT, S., NEWSON, J. and NEWSON, E. (1970). *The Family and the Handicapped Child*. Allen and Unwin.

HICKFORD, J. (1977). *I Never Walked Alone*. Michael Joseph.

HILL, A. (1976). *Closed World of Love*. Shepheard-Walwyn.

HITCHFIELD, E. (1973). *In Search of Promise*. Longman in association with the National Children's Bureau.

HOLMAN, R. (ed.) (1970). *Socially Deprived Families in Britain*. Bedford Square Press.

HOLMAN, R. (1972). *Unsupported Mothers*, 2nd ed. Mothers in Action.

HOLMAN, R. (1973). *Trading in Children*. Routledge and Kegan Paul.

HOTYAT, F. (1974). How children learn new skills. *Advances in Educational Psychology*, **2**. M. L. Kellmer Pringle and V. P. Varmer (eds.), University of London Press.

HUDSON, L. (1972). *The Cult of the Fact*. Jonathan Cape.

HUGHES, A. (1967). The battered baby syndrome. *Case Conference*, **14** (8), 304–8.

HUSÉEN, T. (1974). The purpose of futurologic studies in education. *Advances in Educational Psychology*, **2**. M. L. Kellmer Pringle and V. P. Varma (eds.), University of London Press.

HUTCHISON, D., PROSSER, H. and WEDGE, P. (1979). Prediction of educational failure. *Educational Studies*, **5** (1).

HYMAN, C. (1980). Families who injure their children. *Psychological Approaches to Child Abuse*, N. Frude (ed.), Batsford.

HYMAN, H. H., WRIGHT, C. R. and REED, J. S. (1975). *The Enduring Effects of Education*. Chicago University Press.

JACKA, A. (1973). *Adoption in Brief. Research and other Literature in the United States, Canada and Great Britain, 1966–72; an annotated bibliography*. N.F.E.R., Slough, for National Children's Bureau.

JACKSON, B. and JACKSON, J. (1979). *Childminder: a study in action research*. Routledge and Kegan Paul.

JAFFEE, B. and FANSHEL, D. (1970). *How they Fared in Adoption; a Follow-up Study*. Columbia University Press, New York.

JARUS, A., MARCUS, J., OREN, J. and RAPAPORT, C. (1970). *Children and Families in Israel*. Gordon and Breach, New York.

JENCKS, C. et al. (1973). *Inequality: A Re-assessment of the Effect of Family and Schooling in America*. Allen Lane.

JENSEN, A. R. (1969). How much can we boost I.Q. and scholastic achievement? *Harvard Educational Review*, **39** (1), 1–123.

JOBLING, M. (1977). *The Abused Child: an annotated bibliography*. National Children's Bureau.

JONES, K. (1973). Notes: social work. *New Society*, 1 March, **23** (543), 478.

JONES, K. and FOWLES, A.J. (1984). *Ideas on Institutions: Analysing the Literature of Long-term Care and Custody*. Routledge and Kegan Paul.

JOSEPH, A. and PARFIT, J. (1972). *Playgroups in an Area of Social Need*. N.F.E.R., Slough, for National Children's Bureau.

KAGAN, J. (1970). On class differences and early development. *Education of the Infant and Young Child*. V. H. Denenberg (ed.), Academic Press.

KAGAN, J. (1971). *Change and Continuity in Infancy*. John Wiley, New York.

KAGAN, J. and MOSS, H. (1962). *Birth to Maturity*. John Wiley, New York.

KAHN, A. J. (1969a). *Studies in Social Policy and Planning*. Russell Sage Foundation, New York.

KAHN, A. J. (1969b). *Theory and Practice of Social Planning*. Russell Sage Foundation, New York.

KAHN, A. J., KAMERMAN, S. B. and MCGOWAN, B. G. (1972). *Child Advocacy*. Columbia University School of Social Work. New York.

KAUFMAN, B. N. (1976). *To Love is to be Happy with: the Miracle of One Autistic Child*. Souvenir Press.

KEMPE, R. and KEMPE, C. H. (1978). *Child Abuse*. Fontana/Open Books.

KITZINGER, S. (1969). Communicating with immigrant mothers. *Caring for Children*, M. L. Kellmer Pringle (ed.), Longman in association with the National Children's Bureau.

KITZINGER, S. (1973). Personal communication.

KLAUS, M.H. and KENNELL, J.S. (1982). *Parent–infant Bonding*. Mosby.

KNIVETON, B. H. (1973). The very young and television violence. Paper read at the 17th Annual Conference of the Society for Psychosomatic Research, on 18 October, London.

KOHLBERG, I. (1968). Early education: a cognitive–developmental view. *Child Development*, **39** (4), 1044–55.

KOLUCHOVA, J. (1972). Severe deprivation in twins: a case study. *Journal of Child Psychology and Psychiatry*, **13** (2), 107–14.

LABOV, W. (1971). Variations in language. *The Learning of Language*, C. Reed, (ed.), Appleton-Century-Crofts, New York.

LAING, W. A. (1972). *The Costs and Benefits of Family Planning*. P.E.P.

LAKER, C. and TONGUE, I. (1972). New rights for foster parents. *Concern*, National Children's Bureau (8), 19–25.

LAMB, M.E. (ed.) (1981). *The Role of the Father in Child Development*. John Wiley, New York.

LAMBERT, L. and STREATHER, J. (1980). *Children in Changing Families*. Macmillan, National Children's Bureau Series.

LASLETT, P. (1972). *Household and Family in Past Time*. Cambridge University Press.

LEACH, P. (1979). *Who Cares? A New Deal for Mothers and their Small Children*. Penguin Special.

LEISSNER, A. (1967). *Family Advice Services*. Longman in association with the National Children's Bureau.

LEISSNER, A. (1969). *Street Club Work in Tel-Aviv and New York*. Longman in association with the National Children's Bureau.

LEISSNER, A. (1972). Parents and Children in high-need areas. *The Parental Role*, 22–7. National Children's Bureau.

LEISSNER, A., HERDMAN, A. and DAVIES, E. (1971). *Advice, Guidance and Assistance*. Longman in association with the National Children's Bureau.

LENNEBERG, E. H. (1968). The capacity for language acquisition. *Man in Adaptation, the Biosocial Background*, 2 vols. Y. A. Cohen (ed.), Aldine, Chicago.

LIPSITT, L. P. (1967). Learning in the human infant. *Early Behavior – Comparative and Developmental Approaches*. H. W. Stevenson, E. H. Hess and H. L. Rheingold. John Wiley, New York.

LIPSITT, L.P. (1972). Reciprocating relationships in infant behaviour: congenital and experimental determinants. *Proceedings of the British Psychological Society*, London Conference.

LUNN, J. BARKER. (1970). *Streaming in the Primary School*. National Foundation for Educational Reserach, Slough.

LYNCH, M. A. and ROBERTS, J. (1982). *Consequences of Child Abuse*. Academic Press.

LYNN, R. (1966). *Attention, Arousal and the Orientation Reaction*. Pergamon Press, Oxford.

MACALLISTER, J. and MASON, A. (1972). A comparison of juvenile delinquents and children in care: an analysis of socio-economic factors.

British Journal of Criminology, **12** (3), 280–6.

MCCLELLAND, D. (1973). Testing for competence rather than for 'intelligence'. *American Psychologist*, **28** (1), 1–14.

MACCOBY, E. E. and JACKLIN, C. N. (1975). *The Psychology of Sex Differences*. Stanford University Press and Oxford University Press.

MALLESON, A. (1973). *Need your Doctor be so Useless?* Allen and Unwin.

MALLINSON, V. (1956). *None can be Called Deformed; Problems of the Crippled Adolescent*. Heinemann.

MAPSTONE, E. (1969). Children in Care. *Concern*, National Children's Bureau (3), 23–8.

MAPSTONE, E. (1973). *A comparative study of children in care, based on the National Child Development Study*. Unpublished.

MARJORIBANKS, K. (1978). Family and school environmental correlates of school related affective characteristics. *Journal of Social Psychology*, **106** (2), 181–90.

MASON, M. K. (1942). Learning to speak after six and one-half years of silence. *Journal of Speech and Hearing Disorders*, **7** (4), 295–304.

MAYS, J. B. (1973). Delinquent and maladjusted children. *Stresses in Children*, V. P. Varma (ed.), University of London Press.

MAYS, J. B. (1974). Social aspects of adolescence. *Advances in Educational Psychology*, **2**, chap. 16, M. L. Kellmer Pringle and V. P. Varma (eds.), University of London Press.

MEYERS, E. O. (1973). 'Doing your own think': transmission of cognitive skills from parent and/or paraprofessional to children in the inner city. *American Journal of Orthopsychiatry*, **43** (3), 242–3.

MIDWINTER, E. (1972). *Projections: an Educational Priority Area at Work*. Ward Lock Educational.

MILLER, J. G. (1964). Adjusting to overloads of information. *Disorders of Communication*, D. M. Rioch and E. A. Weinstein (eds.), Williams, Wilkins and Co., Baltimore, Maryland.

MINUCHIN, S. et al. (1967). *Families of the Slum; an Exploration of their Structure and Treatment*. Basic Books, New York.

MONEY, J. (1963). Cytogenetics and cytosexual incongruities. *American Journal of Psychiatry*, **119**, March 1963, 820–7.

MOORE, T. (1972). The later outcome of early care by the mother and substitute daily regimes. *Determinants of Behavioural Development*, F. J. Monks, W. W. Hartup and J. De Wit (eds.), Academic Press.

MOORE, T. V. (1948). *The Driving Forces of Human Nature and their Adjustment; an Introduction to the Psychology and Psychopathology of Emotional Behaviour and Volitional Control*. Grune and Stratton, New York.

MORRIS, P. (1969). *Put Away*. Routledge and Kegan Paul.

MORTIMORE, J. and BLACKSTONE, T. (1982). *Disadvantage and Education*. Heinemann Educational Books.

MORTLOCK, B. (1972). *The Inside of Divorce*. Constable.

MUNDAY, D. (1976). *Dorcas: Opportunity not Pity*. P.H.A.B.

MUSGROVE, F. (1966). *The Family, Education and Society*. Routledge and Kegan Paul.

NASH, R. (1973). *Classrooms Observed*. Routledge and Kegan Paul.

NATIONAL CHILD DEVELOPMENT STUDY USER SUPPORT GROUP. (1985). *Publications Arising from the National Child Development Study*. Social Statistics Research Unit, City University.

NEWMAN, O. (1973). *Defensible Space*. Architectural Press.

NEWSON, E. (1971). Who am I – where do I come from? *Concern*, National Children's Bureau (8) 26–7.

NEWSON, E. (1972). Towards an understanding of the parental role. *The Parental Role*, 28–35. National Children's Bureau.

NEWSON, J. and NEWSON, E. (1963). *Infant Care in an Urban Community*. Allen and Unwin.

NEWSON, J. and NEWSON, E. (1968). *Four Year Olds in an Urban Community*. Allen and Unwin.

NEWSON, J. and NEWSON, E. (1972). Cultural aspects of child rearing in the English-speaking world. *The Integration of a Child into a Social World*, M. P. Richards (ed.), Cambridge University Press.

OAKLEY, A. (1972). *Sex, Gender and Society*. Maurice Temple Smith Ltd.

OFFICE OF POPULATION CENSUSES AND SURVEYS. (1983). *Population Trends* (31), H.M.S.O.

OLIVER, J. E. and COX, J. (1973). A family kindred with ill-used children: the burden on the community. *British Journal of Psychiatry*, **123** (572), 81–90.

OSWIN, M. *The Empty Hours*. Allen Lane, The Penguin Press.

PAGE, R. and CLARK, G. (1977). *Who Cares? Young People in Care Speak Out*. National Children's Bureau.

PARKER, R. A. (1966). *Decision in Child Care. A Study of Prediction in Fostering*. Allen and Unwin.

PARKER, R. A. (ed.) (1980). *Caring for Separated Children*. Macmillan, National Children's Bureau Series.

PEDERSEN, F. A. (1976). Does research on children reared in father-absent families yield information on father influences? *Family Co-ordinator*, October, 459–64.

PFUHL, F. H. (1970). Mass media and reported delinquent behavior: a negative case. *The Sociology of Crime and Delinquency*. M. E. Wolfgang, L. Gavity and N. Johnston (eds.), John Wiley, New York.

PHILP, M. and DUCKWORTH, D. (1982). *Children with Disabilities and their Families*. N.F.E.R./Nelson.

PIAGET, J. (1950). *The Psychology of Intelligence*. Routledge.

PIAGET, J. and INHELDER, B. (1958). *The Growth of Logical Thinking from Childhood to Adolescence*. Basic Books, New York.

PIDGEON, D. A. (1970). *Expectation and Pupil Performance.* National Foundation for Educational Research, Slough.

PILLING, D. (1973). The Handicapped Child. *Research Review* **3**: *Mental and Intellectual Handicap.* Longman in association with the National Children's Bureau.

PILLING, D. (1980). *The attainment of 'immigrant' children: a review of research.* Highlight No. 40. National Children's Bureau.

PILLING, D. and PRINGLE, M. L. KELLMER (1978). *Controversial Issues in Child Development.* Elek Books.

POND, D. A. and ARIE, T. (1971). Services for children in trouble. *Child Care*, **25** (1), 16–20.

PRINGLE, M. L. KELLMER. (1963). 'The happiest day of my life' as judged by junior school children; a longitudinal study. *Current Problems of Developmental Psychology; Festschrift for Charlotte Buhler*, L. Schenk-Danzinger and H. Thomae (eds.), C. J. Hogrefe, Göttingen, Germany.

PRINGLE, M. L. KELLMER (1964). *The Emotional and Social Adjustment of Blind Children.* N.F.E.R., Slough.

PRINGLE, M. L. KELLMER (1964). *The Emotional and Social Adjustment of Physically Handicapped Children.* N.F.E.R., Slough.

PRINGLE, M. L. KELLMER (ed.) (1965). *Investment in Children.* Longman.

PRINGLE, M. L. KELLMER (1966). *Social Learning and its Measurement.* Longman.

PRINGLE, M. L. KELLMER (1967). *Adoption – Facts and Fallacies.* Longman in association with the National Children's Bureau.

PRINGLE, M. L. KELLMER (ed.) (1968). *Caring for Children.* Longman in association with the National Children's Bureau.

PRINGLE, M. L. KELLMER (1969). Policy implications of child development studies. *Concern*, National Children's Bureau (3), 40–8.

PRINGLE, M. L. KELLMER (1970). *Able Misfits.* Longman in association with the National Children's Bureau.

PRINGLE, M. L. KELLMER (1971). *Deprivation and Education.* 2nd ed., Longman in association with the National Children's Bureau.

PRINGLE, M. L. KELLMER (1973). The pre-school comprehensives. *Where* (81), 165–7.

PRINGLE, M. L. KELLMER (1978). A ten point plan for foster care. *Concern*, National Children's Bureau (30), 5–10.

PRINGLE, M. L. KELLMER (1978a). Whither residential care. *Concern*, National Children's Bureau (26), 5–10.

PRINGLE, M. L. KELLMER (1980). *A Fairer Future for Children. Towards better Parental and Professional Care.* Macmillan, National Children's Bureau Series.

PRINGLE, M. L. KELLMER (1981). Towards the prediction of child abuse; Towards the prevention of child abuse. *Psychological Aspects of Child Abuse*, chaps. 11 and 12. N. Frude (ed.), Batsford Books.

PRINGLE, M. L. KELLMER, BUTLER, N. and DAVIE, R. (1966). *11,000 Seven-year-olds*. Longman in association with the National Children's Bureau.

PRINGLE, M. L. KELLMER and FIDDES, D. O. (1970). *The Challenge of Thalidomide*. Longman in association with the National Children's Bureau.

PRINGLE, M. L. KELLMER and VARMA, V. P. (eds.) (1974). *Advances in Educational Psychology*, **2**. University of London Press.

PRINGLE, M. L. KELLMER and NAIDOO, S. (1975). *Early Child Care in Britain*. Gordon and Breach.

PROSSER, H. (1973). Family size and children's development. *Health and Social Services Journal*. (4325 (suppl.)), 11–12.

PROSSER, H. (1976). *Perspectives on Residential Care*. N.F.E.R., Slough, for National Children's Bureau.

PROSSER, H. (1978). *Perspectives on Foster Care*. N.F.E.R., Slough, for National Children's Bureau.

PUGH, G. (ed.) (1979). *Preparation for Parenthood: some current thinking and initiatives*. National Children's Bureau.

PUGH, G. and RUSSELL, P. (1977). *Shared Care: Support Services for Families with Handicapped Children*. National Children's Bureau.

PUGH, G. and DE'ATH, E. (1984). *The Needs of Parents*. Macmillan/National Children's Bureau.

QUINTON, D. and RUTTER, M. (1985). Family pathology and child psychiatric disorder: a four-year prospective study. *Longitudinal Studies in Child Psychology and Psychiatry*, A. R. Nichol (ed.), John Wiley, New York.

RABINOWITZ, A. I. (1969). Co-operation in a multi-purpose school for children aged 2–11 with various handicaps. *Caring for Children*, M. L. Kellmer Pringle (ed.), Longman in association with the National Children's Bureau.

RAYNOR, L. (1980). *The Adopted Child Comes of Age*. Allen and Unwin.

REYNOLDS, D., JONES, D. and ST. LEGER, S. (1976). Schools do make a difference. *New Society*, 29 July.

RIGMOR, EULER VON (1979). The Children's Ombudsman. *IYC/Ideas Forum Supplement*, **10**.

RIST, R. C. (1970). Student social class and teacher expectations. *Harvard Educational Review*, **40** (3), 411–51.

ROBINS, LEE N. (1966) *Deviant Children Grown Up*. Williams and Wilkins, Baltimore, Maryland.

ROSENSHINE, B. (1971). *Teaching Behaviours and Student Achievement*. N.F.E.R., Slough.

ROSENTHAL, R. and JACOBSON, L. (1968). *Pygmalion in the Classroom*, Holt, Rinehart and Winston, New York.

ROWE, J. (1970). The realism of adoptive parenthood. *Child Adoption* (59), 23–9.

ROWE, J. and LAMBERT, L. (1973). *Children Who Wait – a Study of*

Children Needing Substitute Parents. Association of British Adoption Agencies.

RUSSELL, A. (1979). Building concepts through verbal interaction: the key to future success in school? *Carnegie Quarterly*, **17** (1), Winter issue.

RUTTER, M. (1966). *Children of Sick Parents: an Environmental and Psychiatric Study*. Oxford University Press.

RUTTER, M. (1981). *Maternal Deprivation Reassessed*. 2nd ed., Penguin.

RUTTER, M. (1979). Maternal deprivation 1972–1978: new findings, new concepts, new approaches. *Child Development*, **50**, 283–305.

RUTTER, M. and MITTLER, P. (1972). Environmental influences on language development. *Young Children with Delayed Speech*, M. Rutter and J. A. M. Martin (eds.), Heinemann.

RUTTER, M., TIZARD, J. and WHITMORE, K. (eds.) (1970). *Education, Health and Behaviour*. Longman.

RUTTER, M. and MADGE, N. (1976). *Cycles of Disadvantage*. Heinemann.

RUTTER, M., MAUGHAN, B., MORTIMORE, P. and OUSTON, J. (1979). *Fifteen Thousand Hours: Secondary Schools and their Effects on Children*. Open Books.

SANDAY, P. R. (1972). On the causes of I.Q. differences between groups and implications for social policy. *Human Organisation*, **31** (5), 411–24.

SARGEANT, W. (1963). *Battle for the Mind*. Pan.

SCHAFFER, H. R. (1965). Changes in developmental quotient under two conditions of maternal separation. *British Journal of Social and Clinical Psychology*, **4** (1), 39–46.

SCHAFFER, H. R. and SCHAFFER, E. B. (1968). Occasional Paper on Social Administration (25). *Child Care and the Family*, G. Bell.

SCHON, D. (1970). Reith Lectures. Change and Industrial Society. *The Listener*, 19 Nov–24 Dec, **84** (2173–8), 685–8, 724–8, 772–6, 810–12, 835–8, 874–7.

SCHORR, A. L. (1966). *Poor Kids: a Report on Children in Poverty*. Basic Books, New York.

SCHRAMM, W., LYLE J. and PARKER, E. B. (1961). *Television in the Lives of our Children*. Stanford University Press, California.

SCRIMSHAW, N. S. (ed.) (1968). *Malnutrition, Learning and Behavior*. MIT Press, Cambridge, Mass.

SEARS, R., MACCOBY, E. and LEVIN, H. (1957). *Patterns of Child Rearing*. Row, Peterson, Evanston, Ill.

SEGINER, R. (1983). Parents' educational expectations and children's academic achievements: a literature review. *Merrill-Palmer Quarterly*, **29**, 1–23.

SEGLOW, J., PRINGLE, M. L. KELLMER and WEDGE, P. (1972). *Growing Up Adopted*. N.F.E.R., Slough, for National Children's Bureau.

SELYE, H. (1978). *The Stress of Life*. 2nd ed., McGraw-Hill, New York.

SEWARD, J. P. and SEWARD, G. H. (1981). *Sex Differences: Mental and Temperamental*. Lexington Books: Lexington, Mass.

SHEPHERD, P. (1985). *The National Child Development Study: An introduction to the origins of the study and the methods of data collection*. Social Statistics Research Unit, City University.

SHERIDAN, M. D. (1973). *Children's Developmental Progress*. National Foundation for Educational Research, Slough.

SILBERMAN, C. E. (1970). *Crisis in the Classroom: the remaking of American Education*. Random House, New York.

SILVER, H. K. and FINKLESTEIN, M. (1967). Deprivation dwarfism. *Journal of Pediatrics*, **70** (4), 317–24.

SKEELS, H. M. (1966). Adult Status of Children with contrasting Early Life Experience. *Monographs of the Society for Research in Child Development*, **31** (3).

SKINNER, A. E. and CASTLE, R. L. (1969). *78 Battered Children: A Retrospective Study*. National Association for the Prevention of Cruelty to Children.

SKODAK, M. and SKEELS, H. M. (1959). A final follow-up study of one hundred adopted children. *Journal of Genetic Psychology*, **75** (2), 85–125.

SMITH, P. (1980). Shared care of young children: alternative models to monotropism. *Merrill-Palmer Quarterly*, **26**, 371–87.

SMITH, S. M., HANSON, R. and NOBLE, S. (1974). Parents of battered babies: a controlled study. *British Medical Journal*, **4** (5889), 388–91.

SMITH, S. M., HONIGSBERGER, L., and SMITH, C. A. (1973). E.E.G. and personality factors in baby battering. *British Medical Journal*, **3** (5470), 20–2.

SPENCE, J. C. (1947). The care of children in hospital. *British Medical Journal*, **1** (4490), 125–30.

STINCHCOMBE, A. L. (1969). Environment: the cumulation of effects is yet to be understood. *Harvard Educational Review*, **39** (4), 511–22.

TALBOT, N. B., KAGAN, J. and EISENBERG, L. (1971). *Behavioural Science in Pediatric Medicine*, W. B. Saunders.

TALBOT, N. B., SOBEL, E. H., BURKE, B. S., LINDEMANN, E. and KAUFMAN, S. B. (1947). Dwarfism in healthy children: its possible relation to emotional, nutritional and endocrine disturbances. *New England Journal of Medicine*, **236** (21), 783–93.

TANNER, J. M. (1974). Physical aspects of adolescence. *Advances in Educational Psychology*, **2**, chap. 17. M. L. Kellmer Pringle and V. P. Varma (eds.), University of London Press.

TAYLOR, H. F. (1981). *The I.Q. Game: A Methodological Enquiry into the Heredity–Environment Controversy*. Harvester.

TERRY, J. (1979). *A Guide to the Children Act 1975* (as amended), 2nd edn. Sweet and Maxwell.

THORNDIKE, R. L. (1968). Review of R. Rosenthal and L. Jacobsen (*Pygmalion in the classroom*). *American Educational Research Journal*, **4** (5), 708–11.

TIZARD, B. (1977). *Adoption: A Second Chance*. Open Books.

TIZARD, B. (1986). *The Care of Young Children: Implications of Recent Research*. Thomas Coram Research Unit, Working and Occasional Papers 1.

TIZARD, B., MORTIMORE, J. and BURCHELL, B. (1981). *Involving Parents in Nursery and Infant Schools*. Grant McIntyre.

TIZARD, J. (1972). Research into services for the mentally handicapped: science and policy issues. *British Journal of Medical Subnormality*, **18** (34), 1–12.

TIZARD, J. and TIZARD, B. (1971). The social development of two-year-old children in residential nurseries. *The Origins of Human Social Relations*, H. R. Schaffer (ed.), Academic Press.

TIZARD, J. and TIZARD, B. (1972). The institution as an environment for development. *The Integration of the Child into a Social World*, M. P. Richards (ed.), Cambridge University Press.

TOFFLER, A. (1973). *Future Shock*. Pan.

TOLSTOY, L. (1949 edn.). *Anna Karenina*. (Translated by L. and A. Maude), Oxford University Press, World Classics.

TRASLER, G. D. (1960). *In Place of Parents*. Routledge and Kegan Paul.

TRASLER, G. D. (1962). *The Explanation of Criminality*. Routledge and Kegan Paul.

TRISELIOTIS, J. (1979). Growing up in a foster home. *Foster Care*, (19), 12–15, Summer issue.

TUCKEY, L., PARFIT, J. and TUCKEY, B. (1973). *Handicapped School-Leavers: Their Future Education, Training and Employment*. N.F.E.R., Slough, for National Children's Bureau.

VALLENDER, I. (1985). *Education for all: a summary of the Swann Report on the education of children from ethnic minority groups*. Highlight No. 66. National Children's Bureau.

VARMA, V. P. (ed.) (1973). *Stress in Children*. University of London Press.

VERNON, P. E. (1979). *Intelligence: Heredity and Environment*. Freeman.

VYGOTSKY, L. S. (1962). *Thought and Language*. The MIT Press.

WADSWORTH, M. (1979). *Roots of Delinquency: Infancy, Adolescence and Crime*. Martin Roberts & Co., Oxford.

WALKER, A. (1982). *Unequal and Underemployed: Handicapped Young People and the Labour Market*. Macmillan.

WALL, W. D. (1965). The role of education. *Investment in Children*, M. L. Kellmer Pringle (ed.), Longman.

WALL, W. D. (1968). *Adolescents in School and Society*. National Foundation for Educational Research, Slough.

WALL, W. D. (1973). The 'problem' child in schools. *London Educational Review*, **2** (2), 3–21.

WALL, W. D. (1975). *Constructive Education for Children*. Harrap.

WALL, W. D. (1977). *Constructive Education for Adolescents*. UNESCO/Harrap.

WALL, W. D. (1979). *Constructive Education for Special Groups*. UNESCO/Harrap.

WALL, W.D. and VARMA, V.P. (eds.) (1972). *Advances in Educational Psychology*, **1**. University of London Press.

WARD, C. (ed.) (1973). *Vandalism*. Architectural Press.

WARD, C. (1978). *The Child in the City*. Architectural Press.

WEDGE, P. J., ALBERMAN, E. and GOLDSTEIN, H. (1970). Health and height in children. *New Society*, 10 December, **16** (428), 1044–5.

WEDGE, P. and PROSSER, H. (1973). *Born to Fail?* Arrow Books in association with the National Children's Bureau.

WEST, D. J. (1969). *Present Conduct and Future Delinquency*. Heinemann.

WEST, D. J. and FARRINGTON, D. P. (1974). *Who becomes Delinquent?* Heinemann.

WEST, D. J. and FARRINGTON, D. P. (1977). *The Delinquent Way of Life*. Heinemann.

WHALLEY, T. (1973). The needs of the hospitalised child. *Special Education in the new Community Service*: J. W. Palmer (ed.), Ron Jones Publications.

WHITE, A. FRANKLIN (ed.) (1977). *Child Abuse: Prediction, Prevention and Follow-up*. Churchill Livingstone.

WHITE, L. BURTON, KABAN, B.T. and ATTANUCCI, J.S. (1979). *The Origins of Human Competence*. The final report of the Harvard Preschool Project. Lexington Books, D.C. Heath & Co., Massachusetts, U.S.A.

WHITEHEAD, L. (1977). Early parenthood. *Concern*, National Children's Bureau (24), 28–30.

WHITFIELD, R. C. (1980). *Education for Family Life: Towards Preventive Policies for Child Care*. Hodder and Stoughton and National Children's Home.

WILLIAMS, J. M. (1961). Children who break down in foster homes: a psychological study of patterns of personality growth in grossly deprived children. *Journal of Child Psychology and Psychiatry*, **2** (1), 5–20.

WILSON, E. O. (1975). *Sociobiology – the New Synthesis*, Belknap Press of Harvard University.

WISEMAN, S. (1966). Environmental and innate factors and educational attainment. *Genetic and Environmental Factors in Human Ability*. J. E. Meade and A. S. Parkes. Oliver and Boyd, Edinburgh.

WISEMAN, S. (1972). Environmental handicap and the teacher. *Advances in Educational Psychology*, **1**. W. D. Wall and V. P. Varma (eds.) University of London Press.

WITMER, H. L., HERZOG, E., WEINSTEIN, E. A. and SULLIVAN, M. E. (1963). *Independent Adoptions – a Follow-up Study*. Russell Sage Foundation, New York.

WOLFF, S. (1970). *Children under Stress*. Penguin.

WOLFGANG, M. E., FIGLIO, R. M. and SELLIN, T. (1972). *Delinquency in a*

Birth Cohort. University of Chicago Press.

WOOTTON, B. (1959). *Social Science and Social Pathology*. Allen and Unwin.

WYNN, A. (1976). Health care systems for pre-school children. *Proceedings, Royal Society of Medicine*, **69** (5), 340–3.

WYNN, M. (1972). *Family Policy*. 2nd edn. Pelican.

WYNN, M. (1974). *Fatherless Families*. Michael Joseph.

WYNN, M. and WYNN, A. (1973). Using maternity benefits for preventive measures. *Concern*, National Children's Bureau (11), 13–16.

YOUNGHUSBAND, E., BIRCHALL, D., DAVIE, R. and PRINGLE, M. L. KELLMER (eds.) (1970). *Living with Handicap*. National Children's Bureau.

Subject Index